The Modern Polymyalgia Rheumatica Diet

Cheryl White, MA

Sandra Faix, Ph.D.

Contents

THE MODERN POLYMYALGIA DIET

Welcome to *The Modern Polymyalgia Rheumatica Diet*, a comprehensive guide designed to help you manage Polymyalgia Rheumatica (PMR) through the power of nutrition. Living with PMR can be challenging, but by making thoughtful dietary choices, you can reduce inflammation, alleviate symptoms, and improve your overall quality of life. This book is not just about what to eat—it's about how modern concerns such as food allergies, ethical eating, and environmental sustainability can be addressed within a diet designed to combat inflammation.

In the chapters that follow, you will find:

- **An Overview of PMR**: We start by breaking down what PMR is, its symptoms, and how it affects the body. You'll also gain insight into the potential causes and risk factors associated with this inflammatory condition.

- **The Role of Inflammation in PMR**: This chapter explores how certain foods contribute to inflammation at a molecular level and how diet can help you manage PMR by reducing inflammatory responses.

- **Dietary Choices for PMR**: We'll take an in-depth look at different diets such as the Mediterranean and Indian Vegetarian diets, assessing their benefits and how they can be modified for PMR patients. We also tackle ethical concerns, discussing how to make choices that align with personal values while managing the condition.

- **A PMR-Friendly Shopping List**: Learn what to buy, what to avoid, and how to shop smartly for your PMR-friendly diet. We offer suggestions for ethically sourced products and organic options to help you make informed choices.

- **Simple Recipes**: You'll find easy, straightforward recipes that emphasize whole foods, anti-inflammatory ingredients, and plant-based proteins. We keep it simple to ensure you can focus on managing your health, not spending hours in the kitchen.

- **Dining Out and Social Eating**: Practical advice for navigating restaurant menus, making healthy choices while traveling, and enjoying social gatherings without compromising your diet.

- **Personal Stories and Testimonials**: Real-life experiences from individuals managing PMR through dietary changes, offering encouragement and tips that resonate with readers at every stage of their journey.

The Modern PMR Diet addresses not only nutrition but also the importance of modern, ethical eating—considering food allergies, sustainability, and the impact of food choices on the environment. With this book as your guide, you'll find practical, actionable advice for living a healthier life while managing your PMR symptoms.

Let's get started on a journey to better health, balance, and well-being!

1.Why a PMR Diet?

Polymyalgia Rheumatica (PMR) is a condition that involves inflammation, muscle stiffness, and pain, typically affecting older adults. While medication, particularly corticosteroids, is the most common form of treatment, diet plays a significant role in managing the symptoms and mitigating the side effects of long-term medication use.

A well-rounded, PMR-friendly diet can help reduce inflammation, minimize symptoms, and potentially counteract the effects of prolonged steroid use, such as weight gain, diabetes, high blood pressure, osteoporosis, and bruising. This chapter focuses on the critical role of nutrition in living with PMR and how adopting anti-inflammatory dietary choices can greatly improve the quality of life for individuals suffering from this condition.

How PMR Affects the Body

PMR causes widespread muscle pain and stiffness, particularly in the shoulders, hips, and upper arms. This muscle discomfort can severely impact mobility, making it difficult to perform daily tasks like getting out of bed or walking. While the primary treatment for PMR is corticosteroids, these medications come with side effects such as bone loss, weight gain, and an increased risk of diabetes, all of which can be managed or mitigated through a thoughtful diet.

A diet rich in anti-inflammatory foods can help alleviate some of the symptoms caused by PMR and the medications used to treat it. Additionally, by choosing foods that support bone health, maintain muscle function, and reduce inflammation, individuals with PMR can take control of their condition and lessen the physical toll it takes on their bodies.

Causes and Risk Factors

Though the exact cause of PMR is unknown, inflammation is the key underlying issue. Certain factors increase the likelihood of developing PMR, such as genetics, gender, and age. The condition is more common in women and individuals over the age of 50, and there may also be a connection to autoimmune responses or environmental triggers like infections.

Long-term inflammation can contribute to complications, particularly for those on prolonged corticosteroid treatment. Thus, adopting a diet focused on anti-inflammatory foods and nutrients that support overall health is essential.

How Diet Can Impact PMR

A targeted, healthy diet can play a crucial role in managing PMR and preventing complications from medications. By including foods that reduce inflammation and support bone and muscle health, individuals with PMR can enhance their ability to manage the condition.

Corticosteroids, often prescribed to control inflammation in PMR, can lead to side effects such as weight gain, high blood pressure, and bone density loss. An appropriate diet can help mitigate these side effects. For example, including more calcium and vitamin D in your meals can combat bone loss, while reducing the intake of refined carbohydrates and sugary foods can help manage weight and prevent blood sugar spikes.

Nutrients Essential for Managing PMR

1. Calcium and Vitamin D Calcium is essential for maintaining bone health, which is especially important for those with PMR since corticosteroids can cause bone loss over time. Vitamin D aids in calcium absorption, so ensuring an adequate intake of both nutrients is crucial.

Good sources of calcium include:

- Dairy products like milk, cheese, and yogurt
- Leafy green vegetables such as kale and spinach

- Sardines and salmon

- Fortified plant-based milks

Vitamin D can be obtained from:

- Fatty fish like mackerel and tuna

- Egg yolks

- Cheese

- Fortified cereals or breads

- Mushrooms exposed to sunlight

For those who cannot get enough calcium and vitamin D through food alone, supplements are often recommended to maintain bone health and prevent osteoporosis.

2. Healthful Fats Including healthy fats in your diet is another important strategy for managing PMR. Omega-3 fatty acids, in particular, are known for their anti-inflammatory properties, which can help reduce the pain and stiffness associated with PMR.

Sources of omega-3 include:

- Fatty fish like salmon, sardines, and mackerel

- Flaxseeds and chia seeds

- Walnuts

- Fish oils, such as cod liver oil

Including these in your regular diet can help reduce inflammation naturally and may allow for better overall management of PMR symptoms.

3. Anti-Inflammatory Foods Certain foods are naturally anti-inflammatory and should be included regularly to help manage PMR. These foods contain antioxidants and other compounds that support the body's immune system and reduce chronic inflammation.

Key anti-inflammatory foods to incorporate include:

- Leafy greens like spinach, kale, and chard

- Berries such as blueberries, strawberries, and blackberries

- Tomatoes and bell peppers

- Olive oil, particularly extra virgin olive oil
- Nuts like almonds and walnuts
- Fatty fish

By including these foods in your diet, you can help combat the inflammatory response in your body, which is central to managing PMR symptoms.

Foods to Avoid

Just as some foods can help reduce inflammation, others can exacerbate it and should be avoided or limited in a PMR-friendly diet.

Inflammation-triggering foods include:

- Refined carbohydrates, such as white bread, white rice, and pastries
- Fried foods, including french fries and fried meats
- Processed meats like bacon, sausage, and hot dogs
- Sugary drinks, including soda and certain fruit juices
- Alcohol, which can trigger inflammation in the body
- Foods high in trans fats, like margarine and some baked goods

Avoiding or limiting these foods will help keep inflammation levels lower and reduce the severity of PMR symptoms.

Meal Plan Suggestions

Here is a sample meal plan to help you incorporate PMR-friendly foods into your daily routine:

Breakfast:

- Option 1: A bowl of fortified cereal with plant-based milk, topped with blueberries and flaxseeds
- Option 2: Scrambled eggs with smoked salmon on whole-grain toast

Lunch:

- Option 1: Turkey breast sandwich on whole-grain bread with spinach and avocado

- Option 2: Tuna salad with mixed greens, cherry tomatoes, and olive oil dressing

Dinner:

- Option 1: Baked cod with a side of steamed broccoli and quinoa

- Option 2: Grilled chicken breast with brown rice and roasted vegetables

Snacks:

- Mixed nuts (almonds, walnuts)

- Fresh fruit such as apples, oranges, or berries

How Long to Follow This Diet

Managing PMR is a long-term process, and incorporating an anti-inflammatory diet into your lifestyle is a permanent change rather than a temporary fix. Though medication is often essential, especially early in the treatment of PMR, a healthy diet can significantly enhance the body's natural ability to manage inflammation. A diet rich in whole, unprocessed foods is recommended to maintain bone health, manage weight, and control inflammation for life. The dietary changes discussed in this chapter not only help manage PMR but also support overall health and wellness.

In conclusion, the impact of diet on PMR is profound, and thoughtful nutritional choices can make a substantial difference in managing symptoms. By reducing inflammation, improving bone health, and mitigating the side effects of medications, a well-balanced, anti-inflammatory diet is a powerful tool in your arsenal against PMR.

2 The Role of Inflammation in PMR

Polymyalgia Rheumatica (PMR) is primarily an inflammatory condition that causes pain, stiffness, and discomfort in the muscles and joints. While the exact cause of PMR is unknown, it is widely accepted that inflammation plays a central role in the condition. This chapter delves into the connection between inflammation and PMR, explains how certain foods contribute to inflammation at the molecular level, and explores why a low-inflammation diet is essential in managing PMR. Additionally, we'll touch on other diseases that are also linked to inflammation and how they relate to dietary choices.

The Role of Inflammation in PMR

Inflammation is the body's natural response to injury, infection, or other harm. When the immune system detects a problem, it sends out inflammatory cells and cytokines (small proteins that regulate immune responses) to fight off the threat. In cases of acute injury, inflammation is short-lived and resolves as the body heals. However, in chronic conditions like PMR, the immune system's response becomes overactive, leading to ongoing inflammation in the absence of infection or injury.

In PMR, this persistent inflammation targets the synovial membranes surrounding the joints, leading to the characteristic pain and stiffness that patients experience. Although the underlying mechanisms remain unclear, PMR is believed to be linked to an autoimmune response, where the immune system mistakenly attacks healthy tissue, causing chronic inflammation.

One of the biggest concerns with chronic inflammation is the potential for systemic effects. In the case of PMR, inflammation can affect not only the muscles and joints but also the arteries, leading to conditions like giant cell arteritis (GCA), which can cause vision loss or other severe complications.

How Certain Foods Contribute to Inflammation

The foods we eat can have a direct impact on inflammation, either by promoting or reducing it. Certain foods, particularly those high in refined sugars, unhealthy fats, and processed ingredients, contribute to inflammation in several ways.

1. Refined Sugars and Processed Carbohydrates

Foods high in refined sugars and simple carbohydrates (like white bread, pastries, and sugary beverages) can trigger inflammation by causing spikes in blood sugar levels. These blood sugar spikes increase the production of pro-inflammatory cytokines, which are proteins that signal the immune system to initiate an inflammatory response.

Excessive sugar consumption also contributes to weight gain and the development of insulin resistance, both of which can exacerbate inflammation. Chronic high blood sugar leads to the formation of advanced glycation end products (AGEs), harmful compounds that form when protein or fat combine with sugar in the bloodstream. AGEs promote oxidative stress and inflammatory reactions, worsening the inflammatory environment in conditions like PMR.

2. Trans Fats and Saturated Fats

Trans fats, which are found in processed and fried foods, have been shown to significantly increase levels of inflammation. These unhealthy fats activate inflammatory pathways and contribute to the buildup of plaque in the arteries, a condition known as atherosclerosis. This is particularly concerning for people with PMR, as inflammation of the blood vessels is a risk factor in conditions like GCA.

Saturated fats, found in red meats and full-fat dairy products, can also trigger the release of inflammatory cytokines. Although not as harmful as trans fats, excessive consumption of saturated fats can elevate levels of C-reactive protein (CRP), a marker of inflammation that is commonly elevated in people with PMR.

3. Omega-6 Fatty Acids

Omega-6 fatty acids are essential fats found in vegetable oils like corn oil and soybean oil. While these fats are necessary for bodily function, excessive consumption can contribute to inflammation. Omega-6 fats are converted into arachidonic acid in the body, which can then produce pro-inflammatory molecules known as prostaglandins. When omega-6 fats are consumed in disproportionately high amounts (compared to anti-inflammatory omega-3 fatty acids), they promote an inflammatory state.

The Impact of a Low-Inflammation Diet on PMR

Given that PMR is driven by chronic inflammation, adopting a low-inflammation diet can significantly help in managing symptoms and improving overall health. Reducing the intake of pro-inflammatory foods while increasing anti-inflammatory foods creates a balance that supports the body's immune system without triggering excessive inflammation.

1. Omega-3 Fatty Acids

Omega-3 fatty acids are renowned for their anti-inflammatory properties. Unlike omega-6 fats, which can promote inflammation when consumed in excess, omega-3s help reduce inflammation by inhibiting the production of inflammatory cytokines. This makes omega-3-rich foods like fatty fish (salmon, sardines, mackerel), flaxseeds, and chia seeds essential for managing PMR.

2. Antioxidant-Rich Foods

Antioxidants, found in fruits, vegetables, and certain herbs, neutralize free radicals in the body that can cause oxidative stress. Oxidative stress is closely linked to inflammation, and by reducing it, antioxidants help lower overall inflammation levels. Key antioxidant-rich foods include:

- Berries (blueberries, strawberries, blackberries)
- Leafy greens (spinach, kale, chard)
- Nuts (almonds, walnuts)
- Green tea and dark chocolate

These foods help combat inflammation at the cellular level, making them critical components of an anti-inflammatory diet for those with PMR.

3. Fiber-Rich Foods

A diet high in fiber, particularly from whole grains, fruits, and vegetables, can reduce inflammation by stabilizing blood sugar levels and promoting gut health. Fiber supports the growth of beneficial gut bacteria, which produce short-chain fatty acids that have anti-inflammatory effects. Whole grains such as oats, brown rice, and quinoa, along with fruits and vegetables, should be staples in a PMR-friendly diet.

Why a Low-Inflammation Diet Helps PMR

A low-inflammation diet works by reducing the production of pro-inflammatory molecules, supporting immune function, and promoting overall health. By limiting foods that exacerbate inflammation and focusing on those that contain anti-inflammatory compounds, people with PMR can experience reduced symptoms such as muscle pain, stiffness, and fatigue.

Moreover, a low-inflammation diet can help manage some of the side effects of corticosteroids, such as weight gain, high blood pressure, and diabetes. For example:

- Eating more calcium-rich foods like leafy greens and fortified plant-based milks helps protect bone density, which is at risk due to steroid use.

- Including fiber-rich foods helps with maintaining a healthy weight and preventing blood sugar spikes.

- Consuming heart-healthy fats, like omega-3s, supports cardiovascular health and reduces the risk of blood vessel inflammation, particularly in people at risk for GCA.

Other Inflammatory Conditions Linked to Diet

PMR is not the only condition closely linked to inflammation. There are several other chronic diseases where inflammation plays a key role, and diet is a crucial factor in managing them:

1. Rheumatoid Arthritis

Rheumatoid arthritis (RA) is another autoimmune condition characterized by chronic inflammation in the joints. Much like PMR, managing inflammation through diet can reduce pain and stiffness associated with RA.

2. Inflammatory Bowel Disease (IBD)

Conditions like Crohn's disease and ulcerative colitis involve inflammation in the digestive tract. Anti-inflammatory diets, rich in omega-3s and low in processed foods, are often recommended for people with IBD to manage symptoms and improve gut health.

3. Cardiovascular Disease

Chronic inflammation contributes to the development of heart disease, particularly in the form of atherosclerosis. Reducing intake of inflammatory foods, such as trans fats and refined carbohydrates, while increasing omega-3s and antioxidants, can significantly improve heart health.

4. Type 2 Diabetes

Inflammation is closely linked to insulin resistance and the development of type 2 diabetes. A diet focused on whole, unprocessed foods can help manage blood sugar levels and reduce inflammation, lowering the risk of complications.

In Summary

Inflammation is at the heart of PMR, and understanding how certain foods contribute to or reduce inflammation is crucial for managing the condition. By following a low-inflammation diet rich in omega-3 fatty acids, antioxidants, and fiber, individuals with PMR can reduce their symptoms and improve their overall well-being. This dietary approach not only helps manage PMR but also offers protection against other inflammatory conditions, supporting a healthier lifestyle overall.

3 The Science Behind Anti Inflammatory Diets

Inflammation is a natural response by the body to protect itself from harm. In the short term, it helps the immune system respond to injury or infection, facilitating healing and fighting off potential threats. However, when inflammation becomes chronic, it can lead to a range of health problems, including autoimmune conditions like Polymyalgia Rheumatica (PMR). Understanding the molecular impact of certain foods on inflammation is crucial for managing PMR and improving overall health.

This chapter delves into the science behind anti-inflammatory diets, exploring how specific foods and nutrients influence inflammation at the cellular level and why some foods trigger harmful inflammatory responses.

1. Inflammation at the Molecular Level

At the core of inflammation is the immune system. When the body detects harmful stimuli—like bacteria, viruses, or damaged cells—immune cells release signaling proteins called **cytokines**. Cytokines trigger a cascade of reactions designed to neutralize the threat and initiate repair. In a healthy system, once the threat has been dealt with, the inflammatory response subsides.

However, in conditions like PMR, the immune system stays overactive, causing continuous low-grade inflammation. This persistent inflammation damages healthy tissues over time. Chronic inflammation can be worsened by certain dietary choices, leading to flare-ups and increased symptoms of PMR.

2. Nutrients and Phytochemicals that Reduce Inflammation

Certain nutrients and plant-based compounds have been shown to counteract inflammation at the molecular level. These compounds help regulate the immune response, reduce the production of pro-inflammatory cytokines, and promote the production of anti-inflammatory molecules.

- **Omega-3 Fatty Acids**: Omega-3 fatty acids, found in fatty fish like salmon, mackerel, and sardines, are some of the most well-known anti-inflammatory compounds. At a molecular level, omega-3s help by inhibiting the production of inflammatory cytokines like **interleukin-6 (IL-6)** and **tumor necrosis factor-alpha (TNF-α)**, which are commonly elevated in autoimmune disorders. Omega-3s also promote the production of **resolvins**, which actively help resolve inflammation, bringing the immune response to a close and aiding in tissue repair.

- **Polyphenols**: Polyphenols are potent antioxidants found in a variety of plant-based foods, including fruits, vegetables, and spices. For example, **quercetin**, found in onions and apples, has been shown to inhibit the production of inflammatory cytokines like **cyclooxygenase-2 (COX-2)**. **Curcumin**, the active compound in turmeric, similarly downregulates inflammatory markers like **nuclear factor-kappa B (NF-𝜘B)**, which plays a key role in the regulation of inflammation. Curcumin also reduces the release of pro-inflammatory enzymes that are involved in the degradation of tissues, making it especially beneficial for people with PMR.

- **Monounsaturated Fats**: Monounsaturated fats, found in olive oil, avocados, and nuts, also have anti-inflammatory properties. These fats help modulate inflammation by decreasing the production of **reactive oxygen species (ROS)** and reducing oxidative stress, which contributes to chronic inflammation.

- **Vitamin D**: Vitamin D is essential for immune system regulation. Low levels of vitamin D are associated with increased inflammation and autoimmune diseases. Vitamin D influences the immune system by inhibiting the maturation of dendritic cells, which are responsible for presenting antigens to the immune system, and by reducing pro-inflammatory cytokine production.

3. Why Certain Foods Trigger Inflammatory Responses

While some foods help reduce inflammation, others have the opposite effect, promoting the release of pro-inflammatory compounds in the body. This process is often due to the molecular composition of these foods and how the body metabolizes them.

- **Refined Carbohydrates and Sugars**: Foods high in refined sugars and simple carbohydrates—like white bread, sugary drinks, and pastries—trigger a spike in blood sugar. This increase in blood sugar prompts the pancreas to release insulin, leading to an inflammatory response. Over time, chronic consumption of these foods causes insulin resistance, which exacerbates inflammation and increases levels of **C-reactive protein (CRP)**, a marker of inflammation.

- **Trans Fats**: Found in processed and fried foods, trans fats contribute significantly to chronic inflammation. At a molecular level, trans fats increase levels of **low-density lipoprotein (LDL)** cholesterol, which contributes to the buildup of plaque in arteries, causing the immune system to respond as though the body is under attack. This leads to persistent low-grade inflammation. Trans fats also promote the release of **interleukin-1β (IL-1β)**, a pro-inflammatory cytokine linked to conditions like PMR.

- **Omega-6 Fatty Acids**: While omega-6 fatty acids are essential for health, excessive consumption can lead to an imbalance between omega-6 and omega-3 fatty acids, promoting inflammation. Omega-6 fats, found in oils like corn, soybean, and sunflower oil, are precursors to **arachidonic acid**, which the body converts into inflammatory compounds known as **prostaglandins** and **leukotrienes**. The key to reducing inflammation is to balance omega-6 intake with omega-3 intake.

- **Processed Meats**: Processed meats, such as bacon, sausages, and salami, contain **advanced glycation end-products (AGEs)**, which are formed during high-temperature cooking. AGEs trigger oxidative stress and inflammation by binding to receptors on the surfaces of cells. This process activates a pro-inflammatory cascade, increasing the risk of chronic inflammation.

- **Dairy and Saturated Fats**: For some individuals, dairy can be pro-inflammatory due to its high content of saturated fats and specific proteins that may trigger immune responses. Saturated fats found in red meat and full-fat dairy increase inflammation by stimulating the **Toll-like receptor 4 (TLR4)** pathway, which activates immune responses that produce inflammatory cytokines. Individuals with autoimmune conditions like PMR may find that reducing saturated fat intake helps manage symptoms.

4. The Impact of a Low-Inflammation Diet on PMR

By adopting an anti-inflammatory diet, PMR patients can help regulate their immune responses and reduce the severity of flare-ups. A low-inflammation diet works by providing the body with nutrients that support tissue repair, reduce oxidative stress, and modulate immune system activity.

- **Reduced Cytokine Production**: By increasing the intake of omega-3 fatty acids and polyphenols, patients can help lower the production of pro-inflammatory cytokines and increase anti-inflammatory compounds like **interleukin-10 (IL-10)**, which help calm the immune response.

- **Decreased Oxidative Stress**: Antioxidants found in berries, leafy greens, and nuts help reduce the damage caused by free radicals, which contributes to inflammation. By lowering oxidative stress, the body can more effectively manage inflammation without overtaxing the immune system.

- **Improved Gut Health**: Many anti-inflammatory foods, such as leafy greens, fiber-rich legumes, and fermented foods, promote a healthy gut microbiome. Emerging research shows that gut health is intricately linked to immune function, and a well-balanced gut microbiota can help regulate inflammation throughout the body.

5. Other Inflammatory Conditions Linked to Diet

PMR is not the only condition influenced by inflammation. Other chronic diseases linked to inflammation include:

- **Rheumatoid Arthritis (RA)**: Like PMR, RA is an autoimmune condition where the immune system attacks joint tissues, causing pain and inflammation. Anti-inflammatory diets can help reduce symptoms in RA patients.

- **Crohn's Disease and Ulcerative Colitis**: These inflammatory bowel diseases are triggered by immune responses in the gut, and diet plays a significant role in managing flare-ups and promoting remission.

- **Heart Disease**: Inflammation contributes to the development of atherosclerosis, where plaques form in the arteries. A diet high in processed foods and trans fats increases inflammation, while an anti-inflammatory diet can help reduce cardiovascular risk.

- **Diabetes**: Chronic inflammation can lead to insulin resistance, a key factor in the development of type 2 diabetes. Lowering inflammation through diet can help improve insulin sensitivity and manage blood sugar levels.

Conclusion

Understanding the science behind anti-inflammatory diets helps shed light on how specific foods can either contribute to or reduce inflammation at a molecular level. For patients with PMR, adopting a diet rich in anti-inflammatory compounds—while avoiding foods that promote inflammation—can be an effective strategy for managing symptoms and improving overall health. Whether you choose to follow the Mediterranean diet, Indian vegetarian diet, or another anti-inflammatory eating plan, making thoughtful dietary choices is a powerful way to support your body's natural healing processes.

20

4. Ethics and The Environment

When managing Polymyalgia Rheumatica (PMR) through diet, it's important not only to focus on nutrition but also on ethical and environmental concerns. Many people with PMR or similar conditions seek diets that are not only beneficial for their health but also align with their ethical values. For those who have concerns about consuming animal products, especially factory-farmed meat, or want to focus on sustainable and organic choices, several diets can accommodate these preferences while helping to manage inflammation.

In this chapter, we will explore which of the anti-inflammatory diets suit those with ethical concerns, as well as discuss the benefits of organic produce and the potential risks of consuming factory-farmed meat.

Ethical Concerns Around Factory-Farmed Meat and Inflammation

For many, the idea of eating factory-produced meat is not only an ethical concern but also a health issue. Factory farming practices often prioritize profit over animal welfare, leading to overcrowded and inhumane conditions. These practices can raise ethical dilemmas for people who seek to avoid contributing to animal suffering. Moreover, there are health implications associated with factory-farmed meat that could exacerbate inflammation, particularly for people with PMR.

Factory-farmed animals are often raised with the use of antibiotics, hormones, and pesticide-laden feed, which can find their way into the meat. These contaminants can contribute to inflammation and other health issues. For people with PMR, who are already struggling with inflammation, consuming meat that may contain harmful substances like pesticides, antibiotics, or hormones could worsen their symptoms.

Choosing Ethical and Anti-Inflammatory Diets

If ethical concerns are a priority for someone managing PMR, several diets offer plant-based options or alternatives that are more sustainable and ethical, without sacrificing the anti-inflammatory benefits needed to manage the condition.

1. Mediterranean Diet (Plant-Based Adaptation)

The Mediterranean diet is well-known for its anti-inflammatory properties, and it can easily be adapted for those who wish to limit or avoid meat. While the traditional Mediterranean diet includes fish and lean poultry, people with ethical concerns can focus on the plant-based aspects of this diet, such as:

- **Whole grains** like quinoa, barley, and oats

- **Legumes and beans** for plant-based protein

- **Nuts and seeds** for healthy fats

- **Olive oil** as a primary fat source

- **Leafy greens and fresh vegetables**, which are high in antioxidants

- **Occasional sustainable fish**, if it aligns with your ethical stance

For those concerned about the environmental impact of factory-farmed meat, choosing sustainable or wild-caught fish, or opting for organic, pasture-raised meat can reduce the ethical and environmental concerns while still offering the anti-inflammatory benefits.

Benefits for Ethical Concerns:

- Focuses heavily on plant-based foods that reduce inflammation and are sustainable.

- Incorporates healthy fats and proteins from plant sources, reducing reliance on animal products.

- Can include sustainably sourced fish or organic options for those who are comfortable with limited animal products.

2. Indian Vegetarian Diet (With or Without Fish)

An Indian vegetarian diet can be highly beneficial for people with PMR, particularly those who have ethical concerns about consuming meat. This diet emphasizes plant-based foods and can include fish or eggs for those who consume animal products in moderation. The Indian diet also uses spices like turmeric, cumin, and ginger, which are known for their anti-inflammatory properties.

- **Legumes**, such as lentils, chickpeas, and black beans, are a staple in this diet and provide a rich source of plant-based protein.

- **Leafy green vegetables** such as spinach, mustard greens, and fenugreek offer essential vitamins and minerals that reduce inflammation.

- **Spices** such as turmeric, known for its curcumin content, are potent anti-inflammatory agents.

- **Fish**, for those who include it, provides omega-3 fatty acids that help reduce inflammation.

This diet supports ethical concerns by focusing heavily on plant-based ingredients and offering flexibility for those who eat fish or eggs on occasion. Additionally, many of the ingredients used in Indian cooking can be sourced organically, further reducing the environmental impact.

Benefits for Ethical Concerns:

- Emphasizes plant-based nutrition, reducing the need for animal products.

- Rich in anti-inflammatory spices, which can reduce symptoms of PMR.

- Sustainable, particularly if organic produce is used.

3. Vegan and Raw Vegan Diets

The raw vegan diet consists entirely of uncooked, plant-based foods, while a standard vegan diet may include cooked foods. Both diets exclude all animal products, making them ideal for people with strong ethical concerns about factory-farmed meat or animal products in general.

While raw vegan diets can be highly restrictive, a well-planned vegan diet provides many anti-inflammatory benefits through:

- **Fruits and vegetables**: Rich in antioxidants and essential nutrients.

- **Nuts and seeds**: Sources of healthy fats and plant-based proteins.

- **Legumes and whole grains**: Offer fiber, protein, and key vitamins.

- **Cold-pressed oils**, such as olive oil or flaxseed oil, add healthy fats.

However, it is crucial to note that people with PMR on a vegan diet may need to supplement certain nutrients, such as vitamin D, vitamin B12, and calcium, which are harder to obtain through plant-based sources alone. Vegan diets can work well for reducing inflammation, but care must be taken to ensure a balanced intake of all essential nutrients.

Benefits for Ethical Concerns:

- Completely eliminates animal products, aligning with ethical vegan principles.

- Focuses on whole, nutrient-rich plant foods that naturally reduce inflammation.

- Supports sustainability by reducing reliance on factory farming.

Potential Drawbacks:

- May require supplementation of key nutrients such as vitamin D, B12, and calcium.

- Needs careful planning to ensure sufficient protein and healthy fats, especially for people on corticosteroids, who are prone to bone loss.

The Role of Organic and Sustainable Produce

Opting for organic produce can further reduce inflammation and align with ethical considerations. Organic foods are grown without synthetic pesticides, herbicides, or chemical fertilizers, which are known to cause health issues and potentially increase inflammation. Organic farming is also better for the environment, as it promotes soil health, biodiversity, and reduces water contamination.

Choosing organic or locally sourced fruits and vegetables can minimize exposure to pesticide residues, which may contribute to inflammation in the body. For people with PMR, incorporating organic produce into their diet could help alleviate symptoms by reducing these environmental toxins.

Additionally, organic or pasture-raised meats are preferable to factory-farmed alternatives. Factory-farmed animals are often fed grains treated with pesticides, and the animals themselves may be given antibiotics or hormones that can negatively impact human health. These substances can contribute to inflammation, further complicating conditions like PMR.

Benefits of Organic and Sustainable Produce:

- Reduces exposure to pesticides and chemicals that may exacerbate inflammation.

- Supports ethical and environmental values by reducing harm to ecosystems and promoting sustainability.

- Offers cleaner, more nutrient-dense foods that can help improve overall health.

Ethical Concerns with Other Diets

Paleo Diet

The Paleo diet, often referred to as the "caveman" or "stone-age" diet, is based on the idea of eating the foods that our ancestors might have consumed during the Paleolithic era. This means a diet rich in meat, fish, fruits, vegetables, nuts, and seeds while avoiding grains, legumes, processed foods, and dairy. While the Paleo diet has gained popularity for its emphasis on whole foods, it has also raised concerns, particularly regarding the long-term health effects of such a meat-heavy diet.

Potential Health Risks and Concerns

While some people find the Paleo diet beneficial for managing weight or improving energy levels, healthcare professionals have raised concerns about its sustainability and potential health risks, particularly when it comes to cardiovascular health. The diet's high reliance on animal protein, especially red meat, can increase the intake of saturated fats. Saturated fat, in excess, has been linked to an increased risk of heart disease, as it can raise LDL (bad) cholesterol levels.

The Mayo Clinic has warned that while the Paleo diet encourages the consumption of whole foods and eliminates processed foods, it may not be ideal for heart health, especially if followers rely heavily on red meats and animal fats. A diet high in saturated fats and cholesterol from animal products could contribute to the development of heart disease over time, which is especially concerning for people with pre-existing inflammatory conditions like Polymyalgia Rheumatica (PMR), as inflammation and heart disease are often closely related.

Ethical Concerns

For those concerned about the environmental and ethical impact of consuming large quantities of meat, the Paleo diet can be challenging. Factory-farmed meats can contribute to environmental degradation and animal welfare issues. However, some Paleo followers mitigate these concerns by sourcing meat from sustainable, ethical farms that prioritize animal welfare, regenerative agriculture, and low environmental impact.

Balancing Plant-Based Options

One way to make the Paleo diet more ethical and health-conscious is by increasing the intake of plant-based foods that fit within the diet's guidelines. Incorporating more vegetables, fruits, seeds, and nuts can not only improve the nutritional profile of the diet but also reduce the reliance on animal products, helping to lower the intake of saturated fats and cholesterol. For example, using avocados, olive oil, and nuts as primary fat sources instead of animal fats can help reduce the risk of heart disease while staying true to Paleo principles.

Exclusion of Grains and Legumes

Another major criticism of the Paleo diet is its exclusion of grains and legumes, which are not only environmentally friendly crops but also provide important nutrients like fiber, vitamins, and minerals. These foods have been shown to reduce the risk of chronic diseases like heart disease and diabetes, in part due to their high fiber content and beneficial effects on gut health. By excluding these foods, followers of the Paleo diet may miss out on essential nutrients that can help reduce inflammation and promote long-term health.

Potential Drawbacks of the Paleo Diet:

- **Increased Risk of Heart Disease**: A diet high in red and processed meats can increase saturated fat intake, raising the risk of cardiovascular issues over time.

- **Nutrient Deficiencies**: Excluding whole grains and legumes can lead to a deficiency in fiber, certain vitamins (like B vitamins), and minerals such as magnesium, which are crucial for overall health and reducing inflammation.

- **Environmental Impact**: Heavy reliance on animal products, particularly factory-farmed meat, can increase the environmental footprint of the diet unless sourced from sustainable and ethical farms.

: Is Paleo Right for PMR?

For people with PMR, an anti-inflammatory diet is crucial to managing symptoms and reducing overall inflammation in the body. While the Paleo diet can be tailored to focus on whole, nutrient-dense foods, its heavy reliance on meat—particularly red meat—raises concerns about its long-term impact on heart health and inflammation. For those who are interested in the Paleo approach but want to reduce the intake of animal products, incorporating more plant-based, Paleo-friendly options can help make the diet healthier and more sustainable. Additionally, sourcing meat from ethical and sustainable farms can alleviate some ethical concerns.

In summary, while the Paleo diet has its benefits, especially with its focus on eliminating processed foods, it should be approached with caution, particularly for those with cardiovascular risk factors or ethical concerns. It is essential to balance the diet with plant-based foods and healthy fats while minimizing the intake of red meats to reduce the risk of heart disease and inflammation.

For those living with PMR and ethical concerns about their diet, both the **Mediterranean** and **Indian vegetarian** diets offer highly beneficial options. According to the Mayo Clinic, the Mediterranean diet is one of the healthiest approaches to eating, focusing on whole grains, fruits, vegetables, nuts, seeds, and healthy fats like olive oil. The inclusion of sustainable, wild-caught fish provides vital omega-3 fatty acids, which help to reduce inflammation, an essential factor for managing PMR symptoms.

Similarly, the Indian vegetarian diet, which is rich in plant-based proteins from legumes, lentils, and vegetables, provides a variety of anti-inflammatory benefits. The focus on plant-based foods aligns with the ethical concerns many have about factory farming and its environmental impact. Both diets can be adapted to further enhance sustainability by choosing organic, locally-sourced produce and avoiding processed foods.

For individuals with ethical concerns about consuming meat or animal products, these diets offer the flexibility to prioritize sustainably sourced or plant-based alternatives. Incorporating organic produce, responsibly raised poultry, and ethically sourced seafood into these diets can further support both personal health and environmental sustainability. This balanced approach allows individuals with PMR to manage their condition through diet while aligning their eating habits with their values.

In conclusion, the diet you choose to manage PMR should align with both your health needs and ethical values. By selecting plant-based or ethically sourced foods, and by opting for organic produce, you can reduce inflammation while supporting a healthier planet. Let's take a closer look at the Mediterranean and Indian vegetarian diet.

The Mediterranean diet is widely regarded as one of the healthiest dietary patterns, known for its role in reducing cardiovascular disease, promoting longevity, and supporting overall health. Its emphasis on fruits, vegetables, whole grains, healthy fats, and lean proteins aligns well with the nutritional needs of people with Polymyalgia Rheumatica (PMR). However, for those living with PMR, the diet may need some modifications to maximize its anti-inflammatory potential. Additionally, ethical considerations around food sourcing, especially regarding animal products, should be taken into account.

In this chapter, we will explore how to adapt the Mediterranean diet to reduce inflammation in PMR while also respecting ethical choices related to food sourcing and sustainability. This includes focusing on plant-based alternatives, organic produce, and ethically raised animals.

Key Principles of the Mediterranean Diet

The traditional Mediterranean diet is built around the following key components:

1. **Fruits and Vegetables**: Rich in antioxidants, vitamins, and minerals.

2. **Whole Grains**: Staples include barley, farro, bulgur, and whole wheat.

3. **Healthy Fats**: Olive oil, nuts, and seeds are the main sources of fat.

4. **Ethically Raised Proteins**: Primarily fish, with moderate consumption of poultry, dairy, and plant-based proteins.

5. **Legumes**: Lentils, chickpeas, and beans for plant-based protein.

6. **Herbs and Spices**: Flavorful alternatives to salt.

7. **Moderate Wine Consumption**: Red wine in moderation, typically with meals.

Modifying the Mediterranean Diet for PMR

Although the Mediterranean diet has many anti-inflammatory components, certain foods can increase inflammation or may not align with ethical food choices. Here's how to modify the diet for both reducing inflammation and honoring ethical concerns.

1. Whole Grains vs. Refined Grains

The traditional Mediterranean diet encourages the consumption of whole grains, which are high in fiber and help control blood sugar. However, modern variations may include refined grains like white bread and pasta, which can increase inflammation.

Avoid:

- White bread, white pasta, and other refined grains.

Instead, focus on:

- Whole grains like barley, bulgur, farro, quinoa, and whole wheat bread.

- Brown and wild rice, which are rich in fiber and nutrients, helping to keep blood sugar levels stable.

Whole grains are not only beneficial for reducing inflammation but are also more sustainable for the environment compared to heavily processed foods.

2. Dairy Products: Opt for Organic and Plant-Based Alternatives

Dairy is consumed in moderation in the Mediterranean diet. However, some dairy products, especially when not organic or ethically sourced, may contain hormones and antibiotics that contribute to inflammation.

Avoid:

• Non-organic, full-fat dairy, which may contain saturated fats and chemicals that exacerbate inflammation.

Instead, focus on:

• Organic, grass-fed dairy products that are free from hormones and antibiotics.

• Plant-based dairy alternatives, such as almond milk, flax milk, and soy milk, which are often fortified with calcium and vitamin D, essential for bone health in people with PMR.

Plant-based dairy alternatives not only reduce inflammation but also support ethical farming practices by avoiding the industrial farming of animals.

3. Ethical Protein Sources: Focus on Fish and Plant-Based Alternatives

The Mediterranean diet traditionally emphasizes fish as the primary source of protein, with moderate poultry consumption. However, many people with ethical concerns avoid factory-farmed poultry, which is raised in poor conditions that involve cruelty, the use of antibiotics, and environmental degradation.

Avoid:

• Factory-farmed poultry and red meat, which contribute to both inflammation and environmental harm.

Instead, focus on:

• **Sustainably sourced fish**: Fatty fish like wild-caught salmon, sardines, and mackerel are rich in omega-3 fatty acids, which help reduce inflammation. Look for certified sustainable options.

• **Plant-based proteins**: Legumes, beans, lentils, and chickpeas are excellent sources of protein and are more environmentally friendly. They also contribute to a well-rounded diet with anti-inflammatory properties.

- **Free-range, organic poultry**: If you choose to consume poultry, opt for free-range, organic options to ensure the animals were raised humanely and without antibiotics or harmful chemicals. This ensures you are not contributing to factory farming practices.

4. Fats: Prioritize Healthy, Unsaturated Fats

One of the great strengths of the Mediterranean diet is its focus on healthy fats, particularly from olive oil. However, it's important to steer clear of unhealthy fats, such as those found in processed foods and margarine, which can contribute to inflammation.

Avoid:

- Processed oils like corn oil, soybean oil, and margarine.

Instead, focus on:

- **Extra virgin olive oil**: A primary source of fat in the Mediterranean diet, rich in monounsaturated fats that help reduce inflammation.

- **Nuts and seeds**: Almonds, walnuts, chia seeds, and flaxseeds provide healthy fats and are excellent plant-based sources of omega-3s.

- **Avocados**: Full of heart-healthy fats and fiber, avocados also have anti-inflammatory benefits.

By choosing organic oils and sustainably sourced fats, you can minimize your environmental impact while benefiting your health.

5. Processed Foods and Sugars: Limit Consumption

Processed foods, sugary snacks, and beverages are not part of the traditional Mediterranean diet, but they can creep into modern adaptations. These foods are known to increase inflammation and should be avoided for people with PMR.

Avoid:

- Sugary drinks, candy, and processed snacks.
- Refined grains and foods with added sugars.

Instead, focus on:

- Fresh fruits like berries, apples, and oranges, which are naturally sweet and full of antioxidants.

- Using natural sweeteners like honey or maple syrup in moderation.

Sugary processed foods not only contribute to inflammation but often come from unsustainable farming practices. Prioritizing whole, organic foods reduces this environmental strain.

6. Alcohol: Keep It in Check

While red wine, in moderation, is a staple of the Mediterranean diet, alcohol can still trigger inflammation in some individuals. Moderation is key, especially for those managing PMR.

Avoid:

- Excessive alcohol consumption, which can lead to inflammation and other health issues.

Instead, focus on:

- If you drink alcohol, limit yourself to one glass of red wine with meals. Red wine contains resveratrol, an antioxidant with anti-inflammatory properties.

Consider choosing organic or biodynamic wines, which are produced with fewer chemicals, reducing the environmental impact and potential exposure to harmful substances.

Ethical Considerations in Food Choices

For those concerned about the ethics of their food choices, the Mediterranean diet offers a flexible framework. Many people are choosing plant-based diets or reducing their reliance on factory-farmed meats for ethical and environmental reasons. Fortunately, the Mediterranean diet can easily accommodate these concerns:

1. **Plant-based options**: Rely more heavily on plant-based proteins such as beans, lentils, and nuts. A Mediterranean diet based on plants is inherently more sustainable and ethical.

2. **Free-range, organic animal products**: If you do consume animal products, ensure they are ethically sourced. Free-range, pasture-raised animals are treated more humanely and often raised without harmful chemicals.

3. **Organic produce**: Organic fruits and vegetables are grown without synthetic pesticides, which not only benefit your health by reducing inflammation but also help protect the environment by reducing pesticide runoff and soil depletion.

Other Inflammatory Diseases and the Mediterranean Diet

PMR isn't the only inflammatory condition that can benefit from a Mediterranean-style diet. Other diseases linked to inflammation, such as rheumatoid arthritis, lupus, and cardiovascular diseases, also respond well to diets that focus on whole, unprocessed foods and healthy fats.

The anti-inflammatory properties of omega-3s, antioxidants, and plant-based nutrients in the Mediterranean diet make it a powerful tool for managing a wide variety of conditions.

In conclusion, the Mediterranean diet offers a foundation for reducing inflammation in people with PMR, while its flexibility allows for ethical and sustainable choices. By emphasizing organic produce, sustainably sourced fish, and plant-based proteins, you can enjoy the health benefits of this diet without compromising your ethical values. With small adjustments, the Mediterranean diet becomes a powerful ally in managing PMR and improving overall well-being.

In summary, modifying the Mediterranean diet to focus on whole, ethically sourced foods while avoiding processed items and factory-farmed meats can have significant health benefits for those with PMR and beyond. This approach supports both personal health and the planet's health, creating a well-rounded, sustainable dietary plan

6. Indian Vegetarian Diet

The Indian vegetarian diet is deeply rooted in the culinary traditions of India, where vegetarianism is widely practiced due to cultural, religious, and ethical reasons. This plant-based diet, which includes a variety of fruits, vegetables, legumes, grains, and dairy, has become increasingly popular worldwide for its rich flavors and numerous health benefits. For individuals with Polymyalgia Rheumatica (PMR), adopting an Indian vegetarian diet can offer a wealth of anti-inflammatory foods that may help manage symptoms and improve overall well-being.

Understanding the Indian Vegetarian Diet

The Indian vegetarian diet primarily revolves around whole, plant-based foods, with dairy products like yogurt, paneer (a type of Indian cheese), and ghee (clarified butter) also playing key roles. Unlike Western vegetarian diets, the Indian diet incorporates a wide range of spices and cooking techniques that not only enhance flavor but can also have health-promoting properties.

A typical Indian vegetarian meal may include:

- **Whole grains** such as rice, millet, or whole wheat chapati (Indian flatbread)

- **Legumes and pulses** like lentils, chickpeas, kidney beans, and black gram, often in the form of dals or curries

- **Vegetables** including spinach, cauliflower, peas, okra, and eggplant

- **Dairy products** such as yogurt and paneer

- **Spices** like turmeric, cumin, coriander, ginger, and garlic, which add depth to dishes and offer anti-inflammatory benefits

How the Indian Vegetarian Diet Benefits PMR

1. **Anti-inflammatory Properties of Spices**: One of the standout features of the Indian vegetarian diet is its heavy reliance on anti-inflammatory spices. For example, turmeric contains curcumin, a powerful anti-inflammatory compound that has been extensively studied for its ability to reduce inflammation and pain, making it particularly beneficial for PMR patients. Similarly, ginger and garlic have long been known for their anti-inflammatory and immune-boosting properties.

2. **Rich in Plant-based Proteins**: Legumes, pulses, and lentils form the backbone of protein intake in the Indian vegetarian diet. These are excellent alternatives to animal proteins and have the added benefit of being rich in fiber, helping regulate blood sugar levels and prevent energy spikes and crashes. For PMR patients, maintaining stable blood sugar levels is crucial, as high levels of refined carbohydrates and sugars can exacerbate inflammation.

3. **High in Fiber**: A key component of the Indian vegetarian diet is its emphasis on whole grains and legumes, which are rich in dietary fiber. This high fiber intake helps improve digestion and maintain a healthy gut, which is increasingly recognized as an important factor in regulating inflammation throughout the body. PMR patients often benefit from diets that promote a healthy gut microbiome, as an imbalanced microbiome can contribute to inflammation.

4. **Dairy for Bone Health**: Yogurt, paneer, and ghee are commonly consumed dairy products in the Indian vegetarian diet. These foods are rich in calcium and vitamin D, both of which are essential for bone health. For PMR patients, maintaining strong bones is especially important, as long-term use of corticosteroids can increase the risk of osteoporosis. The fermented nature of yogurt also supports gut health, which, in turn, can help regulate immune responses and inflammation.

5.   **Variety of Vegetables**: Indian vegetarian dishes often incorporate a wide array of vegetables, providing a rich source of vitamins, minerals, and antioxidants. Vegetables like spinach, okra, eggplant, and cauliflower are staples, all of which are high in nutrients that support the body's natural defense mechanisms against inflammation. For PMR patients, consuming a wide variety of colorful vegetables helps ensure an intake of diverse nutrients that promote overall health and reduce inflammation.

Ethical and Environmental Benefits

One of the advantages of the Indian vegetarian diet is its alignment with ethical and environmental concerns. Plant-based eating has a significantly lower environmental footprint compared to diets that rely on animal products, particularly factory-farmed meat. By choosing a vegetarian diet, individuals contribute to reduced greenhouse gas emissions and less water and land usage. Moreover, for individuals concerned with animal welfare, the Indian vegetarian diet offers a cruelty-free approach to eating while still providing all the necessary nutrients for good health.

Key Components of the Indian Vegetarian Diet for PMR Patients

1.   **Legumes and Pulses**: Lentils, chickpeas, kidney beans, and other legumes are rich in protein, fiber, and essential nutrients. They help maintain stable blood sugar levels and provide plant-based protein that supports muscle and joint health, which can be particularly helpful for those managing the muscle pain associated with PMR.

2.   **Spices**: The heavy use of turmeric, ginger, garlic, cumin, coriander, and other spices in Indian cooking offers anti-inflammatory and antioxidant properties that may help alleviate PMR symptoms. For example, turmeric's curcumin has been shown to reduce inflammatory markers in the body, offering potential relief from pain and stiffness.

3.   **Vegetables**: Indian dishes often feature vegetables like spinach, cauliflower, peas, and eggplant. These vegetables are rich in vitamins and minerals, including antioxidants that help reduce oxidative stress in the body. By incorporating a variety of vegetables into their meals, PMR

patients can support their immune system and overall health.

4.   **Dairy**: While many Indian vegetarians consume dairy, it is typically from sources like yogurt and paneer, which are rich in calcium and vitamin D. These nutrients are essential for bone health, particularly for PMR patients who may be at risk of osteoporosis due to long-term corticosteroid use.

Modifying the Indian Vegetarian Diet for PMR Patients

While the Indian vegetarian diet is rich in anti-inflammatory foods, certain modifications may be necessary to make it more suitable for PMR patients. For instance:

- **Limit refined carbohydrates**: Some traditional Indian breads, like naan and paratha, may be made from refined white flour. PMR patients should opt for whole-grain alternatives like whole-wheat chapati or millet-based rotis, as refined carbohydrates can increase inflammation.

- **Focus on healthy fats**: Ghee is a common cooking fat in Indian cuisine. While ghee has been shown to have some health benefits, PMR patients may benefit from moderating its use and incorporating more omega-3 rich fats like flaxseed oil or using olive oil for cooking.

In conclusion, The Indian vegetarian diet, with its rich array of plant-based foods, spices, and dairy, offers a balanced and nutritious way of eating that can benefit those with PMR. By focusing on anti-inflammatory ingredients and incorporating ethical and sustainable food choices, PMR patients can help manage their symptoms while enjoying flavorful and healthful meals. With a few mindful modifications, this diet can be a powerful tool in supporting long-term health and reducing inflammation in those suffering from PMR.

Both the Mediterranean diet and the Indian vegetarian diet have the potential to be tailored to gluten-free needs, but each offers different advantages depending on personal preferences and health goals.

Modifying the Mediterranean Diet for Gluten-Free PMR Patients

The Mediterranean diet's focus on whole, unprocessed foods makes it fairly easy to adapt for gluten-free individuals. Here are ways to modify the diet for people with PMR who cannot tolerate gluten:

1. **Whole Grains (Gluten-Free Alternatives)**: Traditional Mediterranean grains such as wheat, barley, and farro contain gluten. For gluten-free individuals, these can be replaced with gluten-free alternatives like:

   o Quinoa

   o Brown rice

   o Buckwheat

   o Amaranth

   o Gluten-free oats

   o Millet These grains are not only gluten-free but also rich in fiber, which is crucial for digestive health and inflammation control.

2. **Avoiding Gluten-Containing Processed Foods**: Many processed foods can contain hidden gluten, particularly in sauces, marinades, and pre-packaged goods. To

maintain a gluten-free Mediterranean diet, ensure that you:

o   Opt for naturally gluten-free whole foods (fruits, vegetables, legumes, and nuts).

o   Check labels for gluten-containing additives.

o   Use homemade or certified gluten-free dressings and sauces.

3.   **Legumes as Protein**: In place of gluten-containing grains, legumes such as lentils, chickpeas, and beans serve as excellent sources of plant-based protein. These can help with inflammation control due to their fiber content and provide sustained energy without triggering gluten sensitivity.

4.   **Nutrient-Dense Fats**: The Mediterranean diet's emphasis on healthy fats, particularly from olive oil, nuts, seeds, and fatty fish, can remain unchanged for gluten-free individuals. These foods are naturally gluten-free and are anti-inflammatory, which helps PMR patients manage symptoms.

5.   **Gluten-Free Bread Alternatives**: While the Mediterranean diet often includes whole-grain bread, gluten-free alternatives such as bread made from almond flour, coconut flour, or other gluten-free grains can be used in moderation. These options can help ensure that you don't miss out on the dietary staples while avoiding inflammation triggered by gluten.

Comparing the Mediterranean and Indian Vegetarian Diet for Gluten-Free PMR Patients

The Indian vegetarian diet, often referred to as "lacto-vegetarian" when dairy is included, is a plant-based diet that incorporates legumes, vegetables, dairy products, and, occasionally, fish. Many Indian dishes are naturally gluten-free, and the diet's focus on spices and anti-inflammatory ingredients makes it an appealing option for managing PMR symptoms. Here's how it compares to a Mediterranean diet for gluten-free individuals with PMR:

Benefits of the Indian Vegetarian Diet for Gluten-Free and PMR Patients

1.   **Naturally Gluten-Free Options**:

o Many traditional Indian dishes are already gluten-free, using grains like rice, millet, and lentils as staples. For individuals with gluten sensitivity, this makes transitioning to an Indian vegetarian diet easier.

o Gluten-free flatbreads like chickpea-based *besan roti* or millet-based *bajra roti* can substitute for gluten-containing breads.

2. **Spices with Anti-Inflammatory Properties**: Indian cuisine relies heavily on spices such as turmeric, ginger, garlic, cumin, and coriander, all of which have anti-inflammatory properties. Turmeric, in particular, contains curcumin, a compound shown to reduce inflammation and pain, which is beneficial for PMR patients.

o **Turmeric**: Known for reducing inflammation and joint pain.

o **Ginger**: Helpful in reducing nausea and inflammation.

o **Cumin and coriander**: Have digestive and anti-inflammatory benefits.

3. **Plant-Based Proteins**: Like the Mediterranean diet, the Indian vegetarian diet provides ample plant-based protein sources such as lentils, chickpeas, and peas, which are also gluten-free and rich in nutrients. These legumes also promote gut health, which may reduce inflammation systemically.

4. **Fish in the Indian Diet**: For those who consume fish, the Indian vegetarian diet can easily be modified to include fatty fish such as mackerel, sardines, and salmon. These fish are high in omega-3 fatty acids, which have anti-inflammatory effects.

5. **Ghee (Clarified Butter)**: Ghee is often used in Indian cooking and is an anti-inflammatory fat that is rich in butyrate, a fatty acid known to support gut health and reduce inflammation. As it is naturally gluten-free, ghee can be an excellent fat for PMR patients.

Challenges of the Indian Vegetarian Diet

- **Dairy Sensitivity**: While the Indian vegetarian diet often includes dairy products like paneer (a type of cheese), milk, and yogurt, some individuals with PMR may be sensitive to dairy or prefer to avoid it. In such cases, plant-based alternatives like coconut milk or almond milk can be substituted.

- **Carbohydrate-Rich**: Some Indian meals can be heavy in carbohydrates, such as rice and lentils, which may not be ideal for individuals managing weight gain from corticosteroid use. Choosing lower-glycemic foods and focusing on portion control can help manage blood sugar levels.

Ethical and Environmental Considerations

For those concerned with ethical food choices, both diets can be adapted to support sustainability and animal welfare. Here are some considerations:

1. **Plant-Based Focus**: Both the Indian vegetarian and Mediterranean diets emphasize plant-based foods, which have a lower environmental impact compared to meat-heavy diets. Eating more plant-based meals also reduces reliance on factory-farmed animal products.

2. **Ethically Sourced Animal Products**:

   o In the Mediterranean diet, it's important to prioritize free-range, organic poultry and sustainably sourced fish to reduce harm to animals and the environment.

   o In the Indian diet, choosing organic and ethically sourced dairy products, as well as opting for plant-based dairy alternatives, supports ethical farming practices.

3. **Organic Produce**: Whether following a Mediterranean or Indian vegetarian diet, opting for organic fruits, vegetables, and legumes is beneficial both for reducing pesticide exposure and supporting environmentally friendly farming practices.

Conclusion

For gluten-free PMR patients, both the Mediterranean and

Indian vegetarian diets offer excellent frameworks for reducing inflammation while managing ethical and environmental concerns. The Mediterranean diet can be modified by focusing on gluten-free whole grains, plant-based proteins, and ethically sourced animal products. The Indian vegetarian diet, naturally rich in anti-inflammatory spices and gluten-free options, is another strong contender, particularly for those looking to emphasize plant-based eating.

In summary, either diet can be adapted to suit personal preferences, health needs, and ethical values, making them versatile options for managing PMR while leading a conscious, healthful lifestyle.

8. Navigating Other Food Sensitivities

Living with Polymyalgia Rheumatica (PMR) is challenging enough, but when you add food sensitivities and allergies to the mix, managing your diet can feel overwhelming. While we've already covered gluten-free options in earlier chapters, there are other common food sensitivities and allergies that individuals with PMR may need to consider. Addressing these sensitivities can help alleviate inflammation and improve overall well-being, allowing you to maintain a balanced diet without triggering adverse reactions.

Understanding Food Sensitivities and Allergies

Food sensitivities and allergies are not the same, though they are often confused. Food allergies involve an immune response to certain proteins found in foods, which can result in severe symptoms like swelling, hives, or anaphylaxis. In contrast, food sensitivities or intolerances do not involve the immune system but can still cause discomfort, such as bloating, gas, headaches, or gastrointestinal issues. Both, however, can exacerbate inflammation in the body and worsen PMR symptoms.

If you suspect a food allergy or sensitivity, it is essential to consult with a healthcare provider or allergist for proper testing and diagnosis. Once identified, you can tailor your PMR diet to eliminate or substitute problem foods while still ensuring proper nutrition.

Common Food Sensitivities and Their Impact on Inflammation

1. **Dairy Sensitivity or Lactose Intolerance**
   - o **What It Is**: Lactose intolerance occurs when the body cannot properly digest lactose, a sugar found in dairy

products. For some, the problem may lie in a sensitivity to the proteins in milk, such as casein or whey.

- o **Symptoms**: Bloating, diarrhea, gas, stomach cramps, and nausea.

- o **Impact on PMR**: Dairy is a source of inflammation for some individuals, especially those with a sensitivity or allergy. Conventional dairy products, especially those from cows raised in factory farming conditions, can be high in hormones and antibiotics, which may further exacerbate inflammation.

- o **Alternatives**: Fortunately, there are plenty of non-dairy alternatives available. Unsweetened almond milk, oat milk, coconut milk, and soy milk can be excellent substitutes for dairy milk. For those seeking calcium and vitamin D without dairy, fortified plant-based milks are a great option. You can also find non-dairy cheeses and yogurts made from almond or cashew bases, and these products can still offer you calcium and probiotics without triggering sensitivity.

2. **Soy Sensitivity**

- o **What It Is**: Soy is a common allergen, and even for those without a full-blown allergy, it can cause digestive upset or inflammation. Soybeans and soy-based products are common in vegetarian and vegan diets, so it's crucial to identify whether soy is a trigger for you.

- o **Symptoms**: Bloating, nausea, fatigue, or skin reactions.

- o **Impact on PMR**: For those with a soy sensitivity, soy-based products like tofu, tempeh, and soy milk may cause flare-ups. Soybeans contain phytoestrogens, which can mimic estrogen in the body and lead to hormonal imbalances or exacerbate inflammation in sensitive individuals.

- o **Alternatives**: If soy is off the table, consider alternatives like pea protein-based products, lentils, or chickpeas for plant-based protein. Hemp seeds and chia seeds are also excellent sources of protein and omega-3 fatty acids, offering anti-inflammatory benefits without the need for soy.

3. **Nut Allergies**

- o **What It Is**: Nut allergies are one of the most common and potentially severe food allergies, particularly to peanuts or tree nuts like almonds, walnuts, or cashews. Reactions can range from mild itching to anaphylaxis.

- o **Symptoms**: Swelling, hives, breathing difficulties, or digestive discomfort.

- o **Impact on PMR**: While nuts like almonds and walnuts are rich in anti-inflammatory omega-3s, they are not suitable for those with nut allergies. Unfortunately, many plant-based products, especially dairy alternatives, are made from nuts, which can limit options for those avoiding both dairy and nuts.

- o **Alternatives**: For those avoiding nuts, seed-based alternatives are excellent. Sunflower seed butter, tahini (made from sesame seeds), and pumpkin seeds are nutrient-dense, anti-inflammatory options that are free from nuts. Chia and flaxseeds can also provide protein, fiber, and omega-3s. Be sure to look for nut-free labels on dairy-free products or explore seed-based alternatives.

4. **Egg Sensitivity**

- o **What It Is**: Some people experience sensitivities to eggs, particularly the proteins found in egg whites. This sensitivity can cause digestive issues and contribute to inflammation.

- o **Symptoms**: Stomach cramps, bloating, skin reactions, or respiratory issues.

- o **Impact on PMR**: Eggs are a nutrient-dense food, but for those with sensitivities, they can increase inflammation and cause discomfort. Eggs are also found in many processed foods, so reading labels is essential.

- o **Alternatives**: For baking and cooking, egg substitutes like flaxseeds or chia seeds mixed with water can act as a binder. Other egg alternatives include applesauce or mashed bananas for baking, and commercial egg replacers are available in many grocery stores. For protein sources, lean meats, fish, legumes, or quinoa can easily replace eggs in meals.

The Role of Organic and Ethically Sourced Foods

Many people with food sensitivities or PMR also express concerns about the quality of their food, particularly when it comes to factory-farmed meat and non-organic produce. Eating organic, ethically sourced foods not only benefits the environment but also reduces your exposure to pesticides, hormones, and antibiotics—substances that can exacerbate inflammation.

1. **Why Organic Matters**: Organic produce is grown without the use of synthetic pesticides, herbicides, or chemical fertilizers. These chemicals can contribute to inflammation and may disrupt the immune system over time. Choosing organic fruits, vegetables, and grains can help minimize exposure to harmful substances, making it easier for your body to manage inflammation.

2. **Ethically Sourced Meats**: If you choose to eat meat, opt for free-range, grass-fed, or organic options. Factory-farmed meat often contains higher levels of inflammatory omega-6 fatty acids due to the animals' grain-heavy diets. Additionally, the stress and living conditions of factory-farmed animals can lead to the presence of stress hormones in the meat, which may negatively impact human health. Choosing ethically sourced meat from animals raised on pasture can reduce these risks.

Tips for Managing Multiple Sensitivities

If you have multiple food sensitivities or allergies, it's important to create a diet that works for your unique needs while ensuring that you're getting all the nutrients necessary for managing PMR. Here are some tips for success:

1. **Plan Ahead**: Meal planning is essential when dealing with multiple sensitivities. Knowing what foods are safe for you and prepping meals in advance can help you avoid accidental exposure to allergens.

2. **Experiment with New Ingredients**: Don't be afraid to explore alternative ingredients, such as quinoa, buckwheat,

millet, or sorghum, to replace common allergens like wheat, soy, or nuts.

3. **Cook at Home**: Preparing meals at home allows you to control the ingredients and avoid hidden allergens often found in processed or restaurant foods.

4. **Label Reading**: Always read labels carefully, especially when purchasing packaged foods. Look for allergen warnings, and be mindful of cross-contamination if you share a kitchen with others who may not have the same dietary restrictions.

Personalizing the PMR Diet for You

Navigating food sensitivities and allergies doesn't have to be overwhelming. By identifying the specific triggers that affect you, you can create a personalized diet that helps you manage your PMR symptoms while avoiding discomfort from other sensitivities. Remember that the key to success lies in balance, ensuring that you are not only avoiding problem foods but also incorporating a wide range of anti-inflammatory, nutrient-dense options.

Whether you're managing lactose intolerance, soy sensitivity, or nut allergies, with careful planning and the right substitutions, you can follow a PMR-friendly diet that supports your health and overall well-being.

9. Foods to Avoid

When managing **polymyalgia rheumatica (PMR)**, understanding how diet affects inflammation is crucial. While including anti-inflammatory foods can alleviate symptoms, avoiding certain foods is equally important, as some can trigger or exacerbate inflammation, making symptoms worse. This chapter will explore key inflammatory triggers and provide guidance on how to recognize and avoid them in your daily diet.

1. Refined Carbohydrates

Refined carbohydrates are often stripped of their fiber and essential nutrients, leading to a rapid spike in blood sugar levels. This can trigger inflammation, which is detrimental for people with PMR, as elevated blood sugar increases the production of pro-inflammatory cytokines. These foods also promote weight gain, which can place additional strain on the joints and worsen PMR symptoms.

Examples of refined carbohydrates to avoid include:

- White bread
- White rice
- Pastries
- Many breakfast cereals
- Crackers made from refined flour

Alternatives: Instead of refined carbohydrates, choose whole grains such as brown rice, quinoa, barley, or whole-wheat bread. These options have a lower glycemic index and provide essential fiber, which helps regulate blood sugar and reduce inflammation.

2. Sugary Foods and Beverages

Sugar is one of the most common dietary culprits for

inflammation. Consuming excess sugar prompts the body to release pro-inflammatory proteins known as cytokines. This inflammatory response can worsen pain and stiffness associated with PMR. Additionally, sugary foods contribute to weight gain and increase the risk of developing metabolic issues like diabetes.

Foods and drinks high in sugar to avoid include:

- Sugary sodas

- Candy

- Baked goods like cakes and cookies

- Sweetened coffee or tea drinks

- Ice cream and frozen desserts

Alternatives: Opt for natural sweeteners such as stevia or enjoy fruit to satisfy sweet cravings. When drinking tea or coffee, try to keep sugar to a minimum, and consider unsweetened beverages like herbal teas or water with lemon.

3. Processed and Red Meats

Processed and red meats have been associated with increased inflammation due to their high levels of **saturated fats** and the presence of **advanced glycation end products (AGEs)**. These are compounds formed when meat is cooked at high temperatures (such as grilling or frying) and can trigger inflammatory responses in the body. In addition, the use of preservatives, nitrates, and other chemicals in processed meats further heightens their inflammatory potential.

Examples of processed and red meats to avoid include:

- Hot dogs

- Salami

- Bacon

- Beef jerky

- Red meat (such as beef, lamb, and pork)

Alternatives: Lean protein sources such as fish, legumes, and ethically sourced poultry (such as free-range or organic options) provide good alternatives. These proteins contain lower levels of inflammatory compounds and offer essential nutrients without contributing to inflammation.

4. Fried and Fast Foods

Fried foods contain **trans fats** and excessive amounts of unhealthy omega-6 fatty acids, which can contribute to systemic inflammation. Fast foods are often prepared using refined oils that are detrimental to overall health, leading to an increased risk of inflammation and exacerbated PMR symptoms. Furthermore, these foods are typically high in calories, leading to weight gain and additional strain on already sensitive joints.

Examples of fried and fast foods to avoid include:

- French fries
- Fried chicken
- Donuts
- Potato chips
- Onion rings

Alternatives: Instead of fried foods, bake or air-fry your meals. For example, you can bake vegetables like sweet potatoes or zucchini for a crispy, nutritious snack. Replace unhealthy oils with anti-inflammatory options like olive oil or avocado oil.

5. Trans Fats and Hydrogenated Oils

Trans fats are a particularly harmful type of fat that increase inflammation, insulin resistance, and bad cholesterol levels. These fats are commonly found in processed foods and certain margarines. They can aggravate PMR symptoms by promoting inflammation in blood vessels and joints, which worsens pain and stiffness.

Foods high in trans fats to avoid include:

- Margarine
- Commercially baked goods (e.g., cakes, cookies)
- Packaged snacks (e.g., crackers, microwave popcorn)
- Fried fast foods

Alternatives: Choose healthy fats like those found in avocados, olive oil, nuts, and seeds. Look for labels that say "trans fat-free" or choose foods that use more natural oils.

6. Dairy Products (for some)

While dairy can be a good source of calcium and vitamin D, it can also be an inflammatory trigger for some people, especially those who are lactose intolerant or sensitive to dairy proteins. Dairy products that are high in saturated fats may contribute to inflammation, potentially worsening PMR symptoms.

Examples of dairy products to watch out for include:

- Whole milk
- Full-fat cheese
- Cream
- Butter

Alternatives: Opt for low-fat or fat-free dairy products, or try plant-based alternatives like almond milk, soy milk, or oat milk. These alternatives often contain added calcium and vitamin D, making them suitable for maintaining bone health without triggering inflammation.

7. Alcohol

Excessive alcohol consumption can increase inflammation in the body by interfering with the body's ability to regulate its immune response. Over time, alcohol contributes to systemic inflammation, which can worsen PMR symptoms. In addition, alcohol interferes with the body's ability to absorb essential nutrients, further complicating overall health.

Types of alcohol to limit or avoid include:

- Beer
- Wine (especially sweet wine)
- Liquor (such as vodka, whiskey, and rum)

Alternatives: For those who enjoy an occasional drink, consider non-alcoholic versions of wine or beer, or simply choose sparkling water with a twist of lime or lemon for a refreshing, inflammation-free option.

8. High-Sodium Processed Foods

High-sodium foods contribute to water retention, which can

cause swelling and inflammation in the body. For people with PMR, this can increase joint pain and stiffness. Processed foods often contain high levels of sodium, along with preservatives and additives that can also contribute to inflammation.

Examples of high-sodium foods to avoid include:

- Canned soups
- Frozen dinners
- Packaged snacks (such as pretzels and chips)
- Processed cheeses

Alternatives: Cook with fresh ingredients whenever possible, and use herbs and spices to add flavor to your meals instead of relying on salt. You can also choose low-sodium versions of packaged foods or rinse canned goods like beans or vegetables to reduce their sodium content.

Hidden Inflammatory Triggers in Packaged Foods

Even when trying to eat a healthy diet, packaged foods often contain hidden inflammatory triggers. Processed snacks, condiments, and even some "health foods" are packed with preservatives, artificial sweeteners, and unhealthy fats that can contribute to inflammation.

Be cautious of:

- Artificial sweeteners (e.g., aspartame, sucralose)
- MSG (monosodium glutamate)
- Added sugars (e.g., high-fructose corn syrup)
- Artificial coloring and flavoring

Reading labels carefully is key to avoiding these ingredients. Opt for whole, unprocessed foods whenever possible, and make meals from scratch to control what goes into your body.

In Conclusion

Avoiding inflammatory foods is a critical step in managing PMR. By recognizing which foods can exacerbate inflammation—such as refined carbohydrates, processed meats, sugary snacks, and trans fats—you can make conscious dietary choices that reduce the likelihood of flare-ups and improve overall well-being. A diet that focuses on anti-inflammatory foods, combined with exercise and stress management, can lead to a more balanced and fulfilling life, even when managing PMR.

This chapter has outlined some of the key inflammatory foods to avoid, offering alternatives that are both nutritious and beneficial for reducing inflammation. Making these changes in your daily routine can go a long way toward reducing symptoms, improving quality of life, and managing the complexities of living with PMR.

Managing Polymyalgia Rheumatica (PMR) often involves a combination of medication, lifestyle changes, and dietary adjustments. While medications like corticosteroids play a significant role in controlling inflammation, supplements can also provide additional support for managing symptoms and reducing inflammation. However, it's crucial to remember that supplements are not a replacement for prescribed medications but can be an adjunct to a well-rounded treatment plan.

Omega-3 Fatty Acids: Nature's Anti-Inflammatory Powerhouse

Omega-3 fatty acids, particularly those found in fish oil, are well-known for their anti-inflammatory properties. In PMR, inflammation is a core issue, leading to pain, stiffness, and fatigue. Omega-3s have been shown to reduce the production of inflammatory molecules, specifically cytokines and eicosanoids, which are responsible for triggering and sustaining inflammation in the body.

Sources of Omega-3 Fatty Acids:

- Fish oil (e.g., salmon, mackerel, sardines)

- Flaxseeds

- Chia seeds

- Walnuts

- Algal oil (a plant-based source of Omega-3)

Benefits for PMR: Including omega-3 supplements or omega-3-rich foods can help lower the inflammation that causes the painful stiffness in PMR patients. It may also help improve cardiovascular health, which is important since corticosteroid use can increase the risk of heart problems.

Considerations:

- Omega-3 supplements can thin the blood, so it's important to consult with a healthcare provider before taking them, especially if you're on blood-thinning medications.

Vitamin D: Essential for Bone Health

Corticosteroid use, while necessary to control PMR symptoms, can have several side effects, one of the most concerning being bone loss. Vitamin D plays a critical role in maintaining bone density and promoting calcium absorption in the body, helping to counteract the risk of osteoporosis associated with long-term corticosteroid use.

Sources of Vitamin D:

- Sunlight (natural production through skin exposure)

- Fatty fish (e.g., tuna, mackerel, salmon)

- Egg yolks

- Fortified dairy and plant-based products

- Mushrooms exposed to sunlight

Benefits for PMR: Supplementing with vitamin D can help protect against bone density loss and reduce the risk of fractures. For those unable to get adequate sunlight or dietary sources, taking a vitamin D supplement may be essential.

Considerations:

- It's important to get your vitamin D levels tested before supplementing, as excessive vitamin D intake can cause toxicity.

Calcium: Protecting Against Steroid-Induced Bone Loss

Since corticosteroids can lead to decreased calcium absorption, it's critical to ensure that PMR patients are getting enough calcium to protect bone health. This is especially important for older adults who are already at risk for osteoporosis.

Sources of Calcium:

- Dairy products (milk, yogurt, cheese)
- Leafy greens (kale, spinach, collard greens)
- Fortified plant-based milk (soy, almond)
- Sardines and salmon (with bones)

Benefits for PMR: Adequate calcium intake helps in maintaining strong bones, reducing the risk of fractures that can occur due to both steroid-induced bone loss and falls caused by stiffness and mobility issues.

Considerations:

- Calcium supplements should be taken with caution and under the advice of a healthcare provider, as excessive intake can lead to kidney stones.

Curcumin: An Ancient Remedy for Modern Inflammation

Curcumin, the active ingredient in turmeric, has been used for centuries in traditional Indian medicine for its potent anti-inflammatory effects. Modern research has supported the use of curcumin as a natural way to help manage inflammation, making it a beneficial supplement for PMR patients looking to reduce their dependency on corticosteroids.

Sources of Curcumin:

- Turmeric root
- Turmeric powder (commonly used in Indian cuisine)
- Curcumin supplements

Benefits for PMR: Curcumin can help reduce inflammation and joint pain, offering relief from PMR symptoms. It also has antioxidant properties, which may support overall health and protect against cell damage.

Considerations:

- Curcumin supplements are not easily absorbed by the body. Look for supplements that include black pepper (piperine), which enhances absorption.

Magnesium: Easing Muscle Cramps and Fatigue

Magnesium is a mineral involved in many bodily functions, including muscle and nerve function. For PMR patients, supplementing with magnesium can help ease muscle cramps and improve energy levels, addressing some of the fatigue that comes with the condition.

Sources of Magnesium:

- Leafy green vegetables (spinach, Swiss chard)
- Nuts and seeds (almonds, pumpkin seeds)
- Legumes (black beans, chickpeas)
- Whole grains

Benefits for PMR: Magnesium can support muscle relaxation, potentially reducing some of the stiffness and cramps that PMR patients experience. It may also improve sleep, which can be disrupted due to pain or corticosteroid side effects.

Considerations:

- While magnesium supplements are generally safe, taking too much can lead to digestive issues, so it's important to follow recommended dosages.

Probiotics: Supporting Gut Health

Corticosteroids can disrupt gut health by affecting the balance of bacteria in the intestines. Probiotics can help restore this balance and support overall digestive health, which is crucial for nutrient absorption and inflammation management.

Sources of Probiotics:

- Fermented foods (yogurt, kefir, sauerkraut, kimchi)
- Probiotic supplements

Benefits for PMR: Maintaining a healthy gut can support the immune system and potentially reduce inflammation, making probiotics a valuable supplement for PMR patients.

Considerations:

- Not all probiotics are the same; it's important to choose a strain that is effective for your needs.

Consulting Your Healthcare Provider

While these supplements can provide numerous benefits for managing PMR, it's essential to consult with your healthcare provider before adding them to your regimen. This is particularly important if you are taking medications for other conditions, as some supplements may interact with prescription drugs.

In Conclusion

Supplements can play a supportive role in managing PMR, especially when used alongside prescribed medications and a balanced diet. Omega-3s, vitamin D, calcium, curcumin, magnesium, and probiotics all offer anti-inflammatory or protective benefits that can enhance your overall treatment plan. By incorporating these supplements mindfully, you can reduce inflammation, protect your bones, and improve your overall quality of life while managing PMR.

62

11 What to Buy at The Store

No matter which diet you follow—whether it's the Indian vegetarian diet or the Mediterranean approach—you'll want to focus your shopping on the outer aisles of the grocery store. The outer perimeter is usually where you'll find fresh produce, lean proteins, and whole foods, which should make up the majority of your diet when managing PMR. Whole Foods, if you're fortunate enough to have one nearby, is a fantastic place to shop. They pride themselves on offering products without additives or preservatives, and all of their fish, dairy, and meat are ethically sourced, making it easier for you to stick to both a health-conscious and ethically-minded diet.

1. Shopping List Essentials

Fresh Fruits and Vegetables

- **What to buy**: Leafy greens (kale, spinach), cruciferous vegetables (broccoli, cauliflower), berries (blueberries, strawberries), tomatoes, cucumbers, peppers, carrots, and sweet potatoes.

- **Why**: Fruits and vegetables are packed with antioxidants, vitamins, and minerals that support your body's natural defense against inflammation. Berries, for instance, are loaded with antioxidants that can help fight inflammation, and leafy greens are rich in nutrients that protect your bones and overall health.

- **Pro tip**: When possible, buy organic fruits and vegetables to avoid pesticide exposure. Not only do pesticides contribute to inflammation, but organic farming methods are more sustainable and better for the environment.

Whole Grains

- **What to buy**: Brown rice, quinoa, oats, millet, farro, and barley.

- **Why**: Whole grains are an important source of fiber, which aids in digestion and supports heart health. Unlike refined grains (such as white bread and pasta), whole grains don't spike blood sugar, which can worsen inflammation.

- **Pro tip**: Look for bulk grains to save money, and store them in airtight containers at home for freshness.

Healthy Fats

- **What to buy**: Extra virgin olive oil, avocados, walnuts, almonds, flaxseeds, chia seeds, and cold-pressed oils like flaxseed oil.

- **Why**: Healthy fats, especially omega-3 fatty acids, have anti-inflammatory properties and can significantly reduce PMR symptoms. Extra virgin olive oil, a staple of the Mediterranean diet, is packed with antioxidants, while avocados offer heart-healthy fats.

- **Pro tip**: Choose cold-pressed, organic oils when possible for the most nutrients and the least amount of processing.

Lean Protein and Fish

- **What to buy**: Free-range poultry, wild-caught fish (salmon, mackerel, sardines), and plant-based protein sources like lentils, chickpeas, and beans.

- **Why**: Protein is essential for maintaining muscle mass, which can be weakened by long-term corticosteroid use in PMR patients. Fish like salmon and sardines are excellent sources of omega-3s, which have powerful anti-inflammatory effects. When buying poultry, always opt for free-range, ethically sourced options to avoid exposure to hormones and antibiotics commonly used in factory farming.

- **Pro tip**: Buy wild-caught fish, as it tends to be higher in omega-3s and lower in contaminants than farm-raised fish.

Dairy and Dairy Alternatives

- **What to buy**: Greek yogurt, almond milk, soy milk, coconut milk, and hard cheeses like parmesan.

- **Why**: If you tolerate dairy, it can be a good source of calcium, which is crucial for bone health, especially if you're on long-term corticosteroids. However, dairy can be inflammatory for some people, so opt for dairy alternatives like almond or soy milk if needed.

- **Pro tip**: Many plant-based dairy alternatives are fortified with calcium and vitamin D, making them great choices for PMR patients who need to support bone health.

Herbs and Spices

- **What to buy**: Turmeric, ginger, garlic, cinnamon, rosemary, basil, and oregano.

- **Why**: Many herbs and spices are natural anti-inflammatories. Turmeric, in particular, contains curcumin, a compound known for its powerful ability to reduce inflammation. Ginger and garlic are also known to boost the immune system and reduce inflammatory markers.

- **Pro tip**: Buy fresh herbs when possible and store them in your freezer to extend their shelf life.

2. Foods to Avoid

To manage PMR effectively, it's just as important to know which foods to avoid as it is to know what to buy. Many processed foods and certain ingredients can trigger inflammation, so here's a list of items to steer clear of:

Refined Carbohydrates

- **Avoid**: White bread, pastries, pasta made from refined flour, and sugary breakfast cereals.

- **Why**: Refined grains are quickly broken down into sugar by the body, causing blood sugar spikes that can increase inflammation and aggravate PMR symptoms.

- **Alternative**: Opt for whole grains like quinoa, oats, and brown rice instead.

Sugary Foods and Drinks

- **Avoid**: Soda, candy, baked goods with added sugar, and sugary fruit juices.

- **Why**: Excessive sugar consumption can increase inflammation throughout the body. Sugary drinks, in particular, can lead to weight gain, which may place extra strain on joints and muscles already weakened by PMR.

- **Alternative**: Satisfy your sweet tooth with fresh fruit, which provides natural sweetness and fiber.

Processed Meats and Red Meat

- **Avoid**: Sausages, hot dogs, bacon, and deli meats.

- **Why**: Processed meats contain high levels of nitrates and other preservatives that can contribute to inflammation. Red meat is also high in saturated fat, which may worsen inflammatory conditions.

- **Alternative**: Opt for plant-based proteins like lentils and beans or ethically sourced poultry and fish.

Fried and Processed Foods

- **Avoid**: French fries, potato chips, and any food fried in unhealthy oils (especially those containing trans fats).

- **Why**: Fried foods contain harmful fats that increase inflammation and can contribute to weight gain and high blood pressure.

- **Alternative**: Choose baked or air-fried options if you crave a crunchy texture, and stick to healthy oils like olive oil for cooking.

Alcohol

- **Avoid**: Beer, wine, and spirits in large quantities.

- **Why**: While moderate alcohol consumption may not have a significant impact, excessive drinking can increase inflammation and interfere with medications used to treat PMR.

- **Alternative**: Stick to water, herbal teas, and natural fruit juices without added sugar.

3. Shopping for Supplements

While it's best to get your nutrients from whole foods, sometimes supplements can help ensure you're getting enough of the essentials. Here are a few key supplements to consider:

Calcium and Vitamin D

- **What to buy**: Calcium citrate or calcium carbonate supplements, vitamin D3 capsules.

- **Why**: Long-term corticosteroid use can weaken bones, making calcium and vitamin D essential for preventing osteoporosis.

- **Pro tip**: Take calcium and vitamin D supplements with food for better absorption.

Fish Oil

- **What to buy**: Omega-3 fish oil capsules.

- **Why**: Omega-3 fatty acids are potent anti-inflammatories and can help reduce PMR symptoms.

- **Pro tip**: If you're not a fan of taking fish oil capsules, flaxseed oil is a great plant-based alternative.

4. Shopping Ethically

When shopping for PMR-friendly foods, consider how your choices affect the environment and animal welfare. Choosing ethically sourced, organic, and free-range options not only supports your health but also promotes sustainability and humane practices.

Organic Produce

- **Why buy organic**: Organic farming avoids the use of harmful pesticides and fertilizers that can not only contribute to environmental damage but also may play a role in increasing inflammation. By choosing organic, you reduce your exposure to toxins and support sustainable farming practices that benefit the planet.

Free-Range, Ethically-Sourced Poultry and Fish

- **Why buy ethically**: Factory-farmed meats often contain hormones, antibiotics, and other additives that may exacerbate inflammation. Free-range and ethically raised animals are treated humanely, and their meat is typically lower in inflammatory compounds.

In conclusion, making thoughtful shopping decisions is essential for anyone managing PMR. Whether you are following a Mediterranean diet, an Indian vegetarian approach, or another health-conscious eating plan, filling your cart with anti-inflammatory, ethically sourced, and nutrient-rich foods is the first step in managing symptoms and improving your overall health

1. My naturopathic physician told me to eat top feeders like salmon rather than bottom feeders like shrimp. Is there any science to this?

Yes, there is science behind the advice to focus on top feeders like salmon rather than bottom feeders such as shrimp. Bottom feeders often live and feed in sediment where contaminants, heavy metals, and toxins like mercury accumulate. Over time, these contaminants can enter the animals we eat and increase the risk of inflammation, exacerbating conditions like PMR. Salmon, particularly wild-caught, is a "top feeder" and is rich in omega-3 fatty acids, which reduce inflammation, making it a better choice for managing PMR.

2. How much fish should I eat if I'm following an anti-inflammatory diet?

For those following an anti-inflammatory diet, it's recommended to eat two to three servings of oily fish per week, such as salmon, mackerel, or sardines. These fish are rich in omega-3 fatty acids, which help reduce inflammation. Vegetarians or those allergic to fish can get omega-3s from flaxseeds, chia seeds, and walnuts, although plant-based omega-3s may be less efficiently absorbed by the body.

3. Are nightshade vegetables really bad for inflammation, and should I avoid them?

Nightshade vegetables (tomatoes, eggplants, peppers, and potatoes) contain solanine, which some believe may contribute to inflammation, though scientific evidence is limited. Nightshades are rich in nutrients and antioxidants that may actually help reduce inflammation. If you notice increased pain or flare-ups after consuming them, it's worth discussing with a healthcare provider.

4. Should I completely avoid dairy if I have PMR?

Not necessarily. Dairy affects people differently. Some find it exacerbates inflammation, while others don't notice any difference. Opt for fermented dairy products like yogurt or kefir, which may reduce inflammation due to probiotics. If you avoid dairy, ensure you get calcium and vitamin D from leafy greens, fortified plant-based milks, or supplements.

5. What's the deal with gluten and inflammation? Should I go gluten-free if I have PMR?

For most people, gluten doesn't cause inflammation unless they have celiac disease or gluten sensitivity. However, some PMR patients feel better without gluten. Focus on naturally gluten-free whole foods like quinoa, buckwheat, and vegetables. Processed gluten-free products often lack nutrients and may be high in sugar or refined carbs.

6. Is organic food really better for reducing inflammation?

While there's no conclusive evidence that organic foods directly reduce inflammation, they tend to be free from synthetic pesticides, fertilizers, and GMOs, all of which can contribute to inflammation. Organic meats and dairy products are also free from added hormones and antibiotics, which may have health benefits. Choosing organic food can be an ethical and health-conscious choice.

7. Can PMR be controlled with diet alone, or will I need medication?

Diet can help manage symptoms of PMR but is typically not a substitute for medication, particularly in the early stages. Corticosteroids like prednisone are often prescribed to control inflammation. Combining medication with a healthy, anti-inflammatory diet may reduce symptoms and lower the need for medication over time. Always consult your doctor before making changes to your treatment.

8. I've heard that turmeric is good for inflammation. How should I incorporate it into my diet?

Turmeric contains curcumin, a potent anti-inflammatory compound. Add it to soups, smoothies, teas, or curries. Pairing turmeric with black pepper increases curcumin absorption. If you don't like the taste, consider supplements, but talk to a healthcare provider first, as turmeric can interact with medications, including blood thinners.

9. How do processed foods contribute to inflammation?

Processed foods are high in unhealthy fats, refined carbohydrates, and added sugars, all of which can lead to chronic inflammation. Processed meats like bacon and sausage contain nitrates and preservatives that increase inflammation. These foods can spike blood sugar and trigger the release of inflammatory markers, making them unsuitable for people with PMR.

10. Can I still have alcohol?

Moderate alcohol consumption, particularly red wine, can have anti-inflammatory effects due to resveratrol. However, excessive alcohol can increase inflammation, interfere with medications, and negatively impact health. If you choose to drink, limit yourself to one glass per day and discuss it with your doctor to ensure it doesn't interfere with your treatment.

11. What about caffeine? Should I cut out coffee?

Moderate coffee consumption doesn't usually worsen inflammation and can even have anti-inflammatory benefits due to its antioxidants. However, excessive caffeine can interfere with sleep, which is crucial for inflammation management. If coffee makes you anxious or disrupts your sleep, consider switching to green tea, which has less caffeine and also contains anti-inflammatory compounds like catechins.

12. What are some go-to snacks for managing PMR on a busy day?

Healthy snacks can help you maintain energy and avoid blood sugar spikes. Some good anti-inflammatory snack options include:

- Mixed nuts (almonds, walnuts)
- Sliced vegetables with hummus
- Fresh berries or other fruits
- Hard-boiled eggs
- Greek yogurt with flaxseeds

- Smoothies with spinach, berries, and chia seeds

13. How important is hydration in managing PMR?

Hydration is crucial for everyone but especially important for those with PMR. Water supports joint lubrication, nutrient transport, and waste removal. Dehydration can worsen symptoms like muscle pain and fatigue. Aim for at least 8 glasses of water a day and increase intake if you're active or in a hot climate.

14. How does stress affect inflammation?

Stress triggers the release of cortisol, which can increase inflammation over time. Chronic stress can also lead to unhealthy behaviors, like poor diet choices or lack of exercise, exacerbating PMR symptoms. Mindfulness techniques, yoga, and regular exercise can help manage stress and inflammation.

15. Are there any foods I should prioritize to help manage corticosteroid side effects?

Long-term corticosteroid use can cause weight gain, osteoporosis, and high blood pressure. To counter these effects, prioritize calcium-rich foods (leafy greens, fortified plant-based milks), potassium-rich foods (bananas, sweet potatoes), and foods high in fiber to maintain a healthy weight and digestive health.

16. Is fasting beneficial for reducing inflammation?

Intermittent fasting has been shown to reduce inflammation in some studies by giving the body a break from digestion and lowering insulin levels. However, fasting may not be suitable for everyone, particularly if you're on medications that require food. Consult your healthcare provider before starting any fasting routine.

17. Are there specific cooking methods that promote an anti-inflammatory diet?

Yes. Opt for steaming, grilling, baking, or roasting instead of frying, which increases unhealthy fats. Using olive oil instead of butter or vegetable oils can reduce inflammation. Also, cooking with herbs like turmeric, ginger, and garlic can enhance the anti-inflammatory effects of your meals.

18. Can sugar substitutes like stevia help reduce inflammation?

Natural sugar substitutes like stevia don't contribute to inflammation the way refined sugars do. However, artificial sweeteners should be avoided, as some studies suggest they may negatively affect gut health, which plays a role in regulating inflammation. When choosing a sweetener, opt for natural alternatives in moderation.

19. Is it safe to take supplements to manage inflammation?

Supplements like omega-3 fish oil, turmeric (curcumin), and vitamin D can help reduce inflammation, but they are not a substitute for a balanced diet. Always consult with your healthcare provider before adding supplements, as some may interact with medications or have side effects.

20. How can I make sure I'm getting enough fiber on an anti-inflammatory diet?

To increase fiber intake, focus on whole grains like oats, quinoa, and brown rice, as well as fruits, vegetables, and legumes. Fiber helps regulate blood sugar, promotes gut health, and can reduce inflammation, making it essential in a PMR-friendly diet.

74

13 Simple Recipes

When dealing with PMR, it's important to maintain a diet that's rich in anti-inflammatory foods while keeping things simple in the kitchen. Below are some easy-to-make, nutrient-dense recipes that are vegetarian-centered with fish options for those who want to include it in their diet. These meals focus on anti-inflammatory ingredients, making them great choices for managing PMR symptoms.

1. Mediterranean Veggie Bowl

This hearty, simple veggie bowl is packed with antioxidants, fiber, and healthy fats. It's also flexible, so you can swap in your favorite veggies.

Ingredients:

- 1 cup cooked quinoa or brown rice
- 1 cup spinach leaves or mixed greens
- 1/2 cup cherry tomatoes, halved
- 1/2 cucumber, sliced
- 1/4 cup kalamata olives
- 1/4 cup crumbled feta cheese (optional)
- 1/4 cup hummus
- 2 tbsp extra virgin olive oil
- Juice of 1/2 lemon

- Salt and pepper to taste

Instructions:

1. Assemble all ingredients in a bowl with quinoa or rice as the base.

2. Drizzle with olive oil and lemon juice.

3. Season with salt and pepper, and mix everything together.

4. Serve immediately and enjoy!

2. Quick Salmon Salad

This is a quick and delicious meal option full of omega-3 fatty acids, which can help reduce inflammation.

Ingredients:

- 1 can wild-caught salmon (look for BPA-free cans)

- 1 tbsp olive oil

- 1 tbsp lemon juice

- 1/4 cup red onion, finely chopped

- 1/2 avocado, diced

- 1/2 cucumber, diced

- Salt and pepper to taste

- 1 tbsp fresh dill (optional)

Instructions:

1. In a bowl, mix the canned salmon with olive oil and lemon juice.

2. Add in the red onion, avocado, cucumber, and fresh dill.

3. Stir gently to combine, then season with salt and pepper.

4. Serve over a bed of mixed greens or in a whole grain wrap.

3. Chickpea and Spinach Stir-Fry

A quick vegetarian meal loaded with fiber, protein, and anti-inflammatory ingredients.

Ingredients:

- 1 can chickpeas, drained and rinsed
- 1 tbsp olive oil
- 2 cloves garlic, minced
- 3 cups fresh spinach
- 1/2 tsp ground turmeric
- 1/2 tsp cumin
- Salt and pepper to taste
- 1/4 cup fresh cilantro, chopped (optional)

Instructions:

1. Heat olive oil in a large pan over medium heat. Add garlic and sauté for 1-2 minutes.

2. Add the chickpeas, turmeric, cumin, salt, and pepper. Stir for 3-4 minutes until chickpeas are warmed through.

3. Toss in the fresh spinach and cook until just wilted.

4. Remove from heat and top with cilantro if desired. Serve with brown rice or as a side dish.

4. Simple Lentil Soup

This easy-to-make soup is rich in protein and fiber, perfect for a filling, anti-inflammatory meal.

Ingredients:

- 1 cup dried lentils (green or brown)
- 1 tbsp olive oil
- 1 medium onion, diced
- 2 carrots, diced
- 2 celery stalks, chopped

- 3 cloves garlic, minced

- 1 tsp ground cumin

- 1 tsp turmeric

- 6 cups vegetable broth

- Salt and pepper to taste

- Fresh parsley, chopped for garnish (optional)

Instructions:

1.   Heat olive oil in a large pot over medium heat. Sauté onions, carrots, celery, and garlic for 5 minutes.

2.   Add the cumin and turmeric, stirring until the vegetables are coated.

3.   Pour in the vegetable broth and lentils. Bring to a boil, then reduce heat and simmer for 25-30 minutes, or until lentils are tender.

4.   Season with salt and pepper to taste. Garnish with parsley and serve hot.

5. Avocado and Sardine Toast

A simple, nutrient-dense snack or light meal. Sardines are a great source of omega-3s, and the avocado provides healthy fats and fiber.

Ingredients:

- 1 ripe avocado

- 1 can sardines (in olive oil or water), drained

- 1 tbsp lemon juice

- 2 slices whole grain or sprouted bread

- Salt and pepper to taste

- Chili flakes (optional)

Instructions:

1.   Toast the slices of bread to your desired level of crispiness.

2.   Mash the avocado in a bowl with lemon juice,

salt, and pepper.

3.   Spread the mashed avocado evenly on the toast.

4.   Top with sardines, breaking them into smaller pieces if needed. Add chili flakes for some spice if desired.

5.   Serve immediately.

6. Berry and Flaxseed Smoothie

A refreshing, antioxidant-packed smoothie that is perfect for a quick breakfast or snack.

Ingredients:

- 1/2 cup frozen mixed berries

- 1/2 banana

- 1 tbsp ground flaxseed

- 1/2 cup unsweetened almond milk (or your favorite plant-based milk)

- 1 tbsp almond butter (optional)

- Ice cubes (optional)

Instructions:

1.   Place all ingredients in a blender and blend until smooth.

2.   Add more almond milk if needed to reach your desired consistency.

3.   Pour into a glass and enjoy!

7. Quinoa and Vegetable Pilaf

A versatile dish packed with fiber, vitamins, and minerals. Perfect as a main dish or side.

Ingredients:

- 1 cup quinoa, rinsed

- 2 cups vegetable broth

- 1 tbsp olive oil

- 1 small onion, diced

- 1 zucchini, chopped
- 1 red bell pepper, chopped
- 1/2 tsp cumin
- 1/4 tsp turmeric
- Salt and pepper to taste
- Fresh parsley for garnish (optional)

Instructions:

1. Cook quinoa in vegetable broth according to package instructions.

2. In a large pan, heat olive oil over medium heat. Add onions, zucchini, and red bell pepper. Cook until soft, about 5-7 minutes.

3. Stir in cumin, turmeric, salt, and pepper.

4. Mix the cooked quinoa into the vegetable mixture. Stir well and cook for an additional 2 minutes.

5. Garnish with fresh parsley and serve warm.

8. Roasted Veggie Salad

A delicious way to get your daily intake of vegetables while enjoying the textures and flavors of roasted veggies.

Ingredients:

- 1 sweet potato, diced
- 1 zucchini, sliced
- 1 red onion, sliced
- 1 bell pepper, sliced
- 2 tbsp olive oil
- Salt and pepper to taste
- 1 tsp dried oregano
- 1 cup mixed greens (spinach, arugula, etc.)
- 1/4 cup feta cheese (optional)
- Balsamic vinegar for drizzling

Instructions:

1.	Preheat oven to 400°F (200°C). Toss the diced veggies in olive oil, oregano, salt, and pepper.

2.	Spread the vegetables on a baking sheet and roast for 20-25 minutes, until they're soft and slightly browned.

3.	Once roasted, place them on a bed of mixed greens. Sprinkle with feta cheese and drizzle with balsamic vinegar.

These simple, anti-inflammatory recipes are great for PMR management. They focus on reducing inflammation while keeping meals easy to prepare. Each recipe can be modified to suit your preferences or dietary needs, allowing you to tailor your diet to best support your health while managing PMR symptoms.

82

14 Fast and Canned Food Options

No matter which diet you follow—whether it's the Indian vegetarian or Mediterranean approach—you'll want to primarily shop on the outside perimeter of the grocery store. That's where you'll find fresh produce, fish, whole grains, and dairy or plant-based alternatives. Stores like **Whole Foods** are great options if available, as they offer products free of additives and preservatives, and all their fish and dairy products are ethically sourced.

In today's busy world, it's not always possible to cook fresh meals from scratch. While homemade, anti-inflammatory meals are ideal, ready meals, fast food, and canned foods are often the quickest solution for those on the go. However, the challenge lies in making smarter choices with these convenient options, especially when managing a condition like PMR, which is often treated with corticosteroids that can lead to other health complications such as high blood pressure.

In this chapter, we'll explore some of the better ready meal, fast food, and canned food options that align with a low-inflammation, PMR-friendly diet. Remember to always be mindful of salt content, as many pre-packaged and fast food options are high in sodium, which can exacerbate high blood pressure. It's crucial to balance convenience with making thoughtful choices for long-term health.

Ready Meals: Healthier, Pre-Packaged Options

1. **Amy's Organic Low Sodium Soups**

   o **Why it's good**: Amy's soups are organic, free from preservatives, and offer low sodium versions. Opt for their lentil, vegetable, or split pea soups, which are packed with fiber and nutrients without the extra salt that can aggravate blood pressure.

   o **Caution**: Even with "low sodium" on

the label, always double-check the amount of sodium per serving. Stick with soups that contain 500 mg or less per serving, and avoid adding extra salt.

2.   **Kashi Frozen Meals**

    o   **Why it's good**: Kashi frozen meals are typically made from whole grains and plant-based proteins. Their meals like the **Sweet Potato Quinoa Bowl** are high in fiber, low in sodium, and feature whole, anti-inflammatory ingredients.

    o   **Caution**: Avoid the varieties that contain processed meats or cheeses, as these can raise your sodium intake.

3.   **Evol Plant-Based Bowls**

    o   **Why it's good**: Evol's plant-based bowls, like the **Butternut Squash & Sage Ravioli**, are packed with fiber and low on sodium, with natural ingredients and no preservatives.

    o   **Caution**: Again, watch the sodium levels. Look for options with 600 mg or less of sodium, which is better for overall heart health.

4.   **Saffron Road Frozen Entrees**

    o   **Why it's good**: Saffron Road offers a variety of meals inspired by global flavors, including vegetarian and seafood options. Their dishes are non-GMO and contain simple, whole-food ingredients. The **Lemongrass Basil Fish** and **Vegetable Pad Thai** are excellent anti-inflammatory options.

    o   **Caution**: Always check the sodium content on any pre-packaged meal. Some dishes can be higher in salt, especially when it comes to sauces.

5.   **CedarLane Frozen Entrées**

    o   **Why it's good**: CedarLane offers a variety of organic, vegetarian, and gluten-free meals. Options like their **Eggplant Parmesan** or **Lentil Soup** are packed with plant-based protein and are lower in sodium than many competitors.

o   **Caution**: These meals can still have hidden sodium, so always compare labels and look for the lowest sodium options available.

Fast Food: Making Smarter Choices

When fast food is your only option, it's easy to fall into the trap of ordering highly processed, salty meals. However, there are ways to choose healthier options even at fast food chains:

1.   **Subway's Veggie Delite Salad**

o   **Why it's good**: Subway offers a variety of fresh salads, and the Veggie Delite can be loaded with fresh vegetables. Avoid adding processed meats and cheeses, and go for olive oil and vinegar instead of salt-heavy dressings.

o   **Caution**: Be mindful of condiments and dressings—many contain added sugars and sodium, which can undo the benefits of an otherwise healthy meal.

2.   **Chipotle's Burrito Bowl with Brown Rice and Veggies**

o   **Why it's good**: At Chipotle, you can customize a healthy burrito bowl by choosing brown rice, black beans, grilled vegetables, and fresh salsas. Skip the cheese and sour cream to avoid extra saturated fats.

o   **Caution**: Chipotle's salsas and rice can still be high in sodium. Ask for less rice and more veggies, and stay hydrated by drinking water when eating out to balance out sodium intake.

3.   **Panera Bread's Mediterranean Veggie Sandwich**

o   **Why it's good**: Panera's Mediterranean Veggie Sandwich is full of vegetables and hummus. You can request whole grain bread for added fiber and ask for less feta cheese to reduce sodium.

o   **Caution**: Panera's offerings are notorious for high sodium levels—even their seemingly healthy options. Ask for no added salt in soups or salads, and remember that soups at Panera often pack more sodium than you think, even with vegetable-based broths. While Panera offers good ingredients, be cautious of the overall salt content in their meals to avoid complications with blood pressure.

4.   **Starbucks Protein Boxes**

o   **Why it's good**: Starbucks offers protein boxes with fresh fruit, hard-boiled eggs, and nuts. These boxes can be a good choice for a quick, balanced meal with protein and healthy fats.

o   **Caution**: Avoid any boxes with processed cheeses or meats, which are often high in salt and unhealthy fats.

5.   **Sweetgreen's Plant-Based Bowls**

o   **Why it's good**: Sweetgreen is known for its seasonal salads and bowls filled with whole, fresh ingredients. Opt for their **Shroomami Bowl**, which contains a hearty serving of mushrooms, wild rice, and tofu—all anti-inflammatory choices.

o   **Caution**: Watch the dressings. Even if a bowl is full of healthy ingredients, the dressing can still carry a lot of sodium or added sugars. Stick with olive oil-based dressings or light vinaigrettes.

Canned Foods: Stocking Your Pantry Wisely

Canned foods are another convenient option, but they often come loaded with salt and preservatives. However, there are healthier options that provide the convenience of shelf-stable items without sacrificing nutrition:

1.   **Wild Planet Canned Salmon or Sardines**

o   **Why it's good**: Wild Planet's products are sustainably sourced and rich in omega-3 fatty acids, which are great for reducing inflammation. These make a great pantry staple for quick, nutritious meals.

o   **Caution**: Opt for canned fish in water rather than oil to avoid unnecessary calories and fats.

Also, check sodium levels—canned fish can be high in salt, so choose low-sodium versions when possible.

2.   **Eden Organic Beans**

o   **Why it's good**: Eden Organic beans are low in sodium and come without preservatives. They are an excellent source of plant-based protein and fiber, which can help reduce inflammation.

o   **Caution**: Rinse canned beans under cold water before using them to remove any excess sodium, even if they are labeled "low-sodium."

3.   **Muir Glen Organic Canned Tomatoes**

o   **Why it's good**: Muir Glen offers organic, BPA-free canned tomatoes, which are perfect for soups, stews, and sauces. Tomatoes are rich in lycopene, an antioxidant that fights inflammation.

o   **Caution**: Check the label for added sugars and sodium, which are common in canned tomato products.

4.   **Amy's Organic Refried Beans (Light in Sodium)**

o   **Why it's good**: These refried beans are light in sodium and packed with plant-based proteins and fiber. They're a good option for quick, healthy meals.

o   **Caution**: As with other canned goods, check the sodium content and avoid products with added fats.

5.   **Pacific Foods Organic Soups**

o   **Why it's good**: Pacific Foods offers a wide variety of organic soups, from vegetable to tomato basil. Their soups are made with real ingredients and without preservatives, making them a solid option for quick meals.

o   **Caution**: Again, always check the sodium levels. Even with organic products, salt can be a hidden culprit. Go for the low-sodium versions whenever possible.

6.   Trader Joe's Canned Lentil Soup

o   **Why it's good**: Trader Joe's canned lentil soup is packed with plant-based protein and fiber, making it a quick, anti-inflammatory option for those short on time. The ingredients are simple and straightforward.

o   **Caution**: While Trader Joe's generally keeps things healthy, the sodium content in canned soups can still be high. Always go for the low-sodium version when available, or consider diluting the soup with water.

7.   BPA-Free Canned Coconut Milk

o   **Why it's good**: Canned coconut milk is a great pantry staple for adding richness to curries, soups, or smoothies. Coconut has anti-inflammatory properties, and BPA-free cans ensure you're avoiding harmful chemicals.

o   **Caution**: Coconut milk is high in fat, so use it in moderation, especially if you are watching your fat intake. Make sure to get unsweetened varieties to avoid added sugars.

While convenient food options are necessary for busy lifestyles, they don't have to undermine your health or exacerbate your PMR symptoms. The key is to read labels carefully, watch your sodium intake, and prioritize whole, nutrient-dense foods. Whenever possible, opt for organic, sustainably sourced options, especially when it comes to fish, poultry, and produce.

Even when life gets busy, you can still make choices that align with your health goals. Pre-packaged meals, fast food, and canned goods can be part of a healthy, anti-inflammatory diet if you choose wisely.

15 Dining Out and Social Eating

For people with PMR, maintaining an anti-inflammatory diet can sometimes be challenging, especially when dining out or attending social gatherings. However, with a little planning and knowledge, you can make choices that align with your dietary needs without feeling deprived. In this chapter, we'll explore how to navigate restaurant menus, prepare travel-friendly snacks, and manage holiday meals and social events with confidence.

Navigating Restaurant Menus

Dining out doesn't have to derail your efforts to maintain an anti-inflammatory diet. With a few key strategies, you can enjoy restaurant meals while still prioritizing your health:

1. **Start with the Basics**: Stick to simple, whole foods whenever possible. Look for menu items that feature grilled, steamed, roasted, or baked options instead of fried or heavily processed foods. These options tend to be lower in trans fats and refined oils, both of which can promote inflammation.

2. **Choose Lean Proteins and Healthy Fats**: Opt for fish, especially those high in omega-3 fatty acids like salmon, sardines, or mackerel. Grilled chicken or turkey can be good choices as well—just be sure to ask if they offer free-range or organic poultry, as these are less likely to be exposed to chemicals that could contribute to inflammation. Avoid processed meats like sausages or deli meats, as they can contain preservatives and high levels of sodium, which can exacerbate inflammation.

3. **Ask for Customizations**: Don't hesitate to ask for modifications. Many restaurants are happy to accommodate

dietary preferences, whether that means swapping out a side of fries for a salad or replacing bread with extra vegetables. Request sauces and dressings on the side, as these can often be high in sugar or unhealthy fats. Olive oil and vinegar is a great alternative to many commercial dressings.

4. **Watch Out for Hidden Sugars**: Be mindful of dressings, marinades, and sauces, which can often be laden with sugar or refined carbohydrates. Tomato-based sauces can sometimes be packed with sugar, so it's worth asking about the ingredients. Instead, look for olive oil-based dressings, lemon juice, or even a simple herb garnish to enhance the flavor of your dish.

5. **Focus on Vegetables**: One of the easiest ways to ensure your meal is anti-inflammatory is to load up on vegetables. Opt for sides like sautéed spinach, roasted Brussels sprouts, or steamed broccoli. Restaurants offering Mediterranean cuisine tend to have a wide array of vegetable-based dishes, so exploring these options can be a great way to stay aligned with your diet while dining out.

6. **Skip Refined Carbs**: Many restaurant dishes come with white bread, pasta, or rice, which are all refined carbohydrates that can spike blood sugar and promote inflammation. Ask if whole grains like quinoa, brown rice, or whole wheat pasta are available as alternatives. If not, consider skipping the carb-heavy portion altogether and focusing on vegetables and proteins instead.

Travel-Friendly Snacks

When you're on the go, having nutritious, anti-inflammatory snacks at hand can help you avoid unhealthy options at convenience stores or fast food chains. Below are some easy, portable snack ideas that align with an anti-inflammatory diet:

1. **Nuts and Seeds**: Almonds, walnuts, flaxseeds, and chia seeds are all great sources of healthy fats and omega-3 fatty acids, which help reduce inflammation. Be sure to choose unsalted, raw, or dry-roasted varieties to avoid added sodium and unhealthy oils.

2. **Fresh Fruit**: Apples, oranges, and berries are easy to pack and offer plenty of antioxidants and fiber, both of which help to

lower inflammation. A small container of mixed berries is perfect for travel, as they are anti-inflammatory powerhouses.

3. **Vegetable Sticks and Hummus**: Carrot and cucumber sticks paired with hummus make a nutritious, filling snack. Hummus is made from chickpeas, which are high in fiber and healthy fats, and the vegetables provide vitamins and minerals without the refined sugars found in processed snacks.

4. **Nut Butter Packets**: Single-serving packets of almond butter or peanut butter (ideally without added sugar) are a convenient way to get healthy fats while on the go. Pair with sliced fruit or whole grain crackers for a more substantial snack.

5. **Hard-Boiled Eggs**: Easy to prepare ahead of time, hard-boiled eggs provide a great source of protein and healthy fats. They are filling and convenient, making them a perfect travel snack.

6. **Roasted Chickpeas**: Crunchy roasted chickpeas are a great alternative to chips or crackers, offering both protein and fiber in a portable form. Season them with anti-inflammatory spices like turmeric or paprika for added flavor and benefits.

7. **Olives**: A small container of olives can be a quick snack packed with healthy fats. They're especially rich in anti-inflammatory compounds like oleic acid, a type of monounsaturated fat that's also found in olive oil.

Holiday Meals and Gatherings

Social events, holidays, and gatherings can be tricky to navigate when you're trying to stick to an anti-inflammatory diet. Here are some tips to help you enjoy these occasions while staying true to your health goals:

1. **Offer to Bring a Dish**: If you're attending a potluck or family gathering, offer to bring a dish that you know fits your dietary needs. You could prepare a large vegetable-based dish, like a roasted vegetable platter, a quinoa salad, or a fish-based entrée, ensuring there's at least one item you can enjoy without worry.

2. **Be Mindful of Holiday Meats**: Traditional holiday meals often include meat, but you can make anti-inflammatory choices by opting for ethically sourced, free-range poultry or sustainably caught fish. Avoid processed meats like ham or bacon, which are high in sodium and preservatives.

3. **Choose Healthier Cooking Methods**: When preparing holiday meals, focus on grilling, roasting, or baking instead of frying. For example, roasted root vegetables like sweet potatoes, carrots, and beets make a great side dish and provide plenty of fiber and antioxidants.

4. **Load Up on Vegetables**: At social events or holiday gatherings, try to fill your plate with vegetable-based dishes first. Roasted vegetables, salads, and sautéed greens are often available, and they can help balance out richer, more indulgent foods.

5. **Stay Hydrated**: Drink plenty of water before and during meals, especially if you're consuming foods that are higher in sodium or you're enjoying an alcoholic drink. Staying hydrated can help your body process foods more efficiently and prevent overeating.

6. **Watch Portion Sizes**: With so many tempting dishes at holiday meals, it's easy to overindulge. Keep your portion sizes moderate, especially for foods that are high in sugar, fat, or refined carbohydrates. Take smaller servings of these items and balance them out with nutrient-dense vegetables and proteins.

7. **Modify Traditional Recipes**: You can make healthier versions of holiday classics by swapping out certain ingredients. For example, use whole grain flour in place of white flour for baking, or substitute olive oil for butter in savory dishes. Instead of sugary desserts, consider serving fruit-based options like baked apples or a berry compote.

In Conclusion

Dining out, traveling, and attending social events while sticking to an anti-inflammatory diet doesn't have to be overwhelming. By making smart choices and planning ahead, you can enjoy meals with friends and family without sacrificing your health goals. Remember to prioritize whole foods, lean proteins, healthy fats, and plenty of vegetables, and don't hesitate to ask for modifications when needed. Whether you're at a restaurant, on the road, or celebrating a special occasion, you can stay on track and feel your best.

16. Patient Stories

Diet plays an essential role in managing Polymyalgia Rheumatica (PMR), but each person's journey with the condition is unique. In this chapter, we share personal stories and testimonials from individuals with PMR who have found success using dietary interventions. These stories illustrate a diverse range of experiences, from those newly diagnosed and grappling with the early stages of the disease to individuals who have been managing PMR for years and have discovered how nutrition can be a powerful tool in their overall treatment plan.

Anna's Story: Adjusting to Life with PMR

Anna, a retired teacher in her late 60s, was diagnosed with PMR after experiencing persistent pain and stiffness in her shoulders and hips. Her active lifestyle suddenly came to a halt when she could no longer garden or walk her dog without wincing in pain. Corticosteroids helped relieve some of her symptoms, but she quickly experienced side effects like weight gain, mood swings, and trouble sleeping.

"I knew I couldn't rely on medication alone," Anna explains. "So I started researching how diet might help. I'd always eaten fairly healthy, but I realized I could do more to reduce inflammation."

Anna adopted a Mediterranean-style diet, focusing on incorporating more fish, olive oil, nuts, and fresh vegetables. She cut out red meat and processed foods and made an effort to cook more at home. Initially skeptical, she started to notice improvements within a couple of months.

"I didn't think food could have such a big impact," she says. "But my energy levels improved, and I started feeling less achy in the mornings. My weight stabilized, and I was able to reduce my steroid dose with my doctor's help."

Anna continues to manage her symptoms through a combination of diet, medication, and light exercise, and she encourages others with PMR to consider dietary changes. "It's not a cure, but it's definitely helped me feel more like myself again."

Jake's Story: Battling the Side Effects of Medication

Jake, 42, works as an IT consultant and was diagnosed with PMR after months of unexplained pain and fatigue. His job requires him to sit for long periods, which made his stiffness even worse. He was placed on corticosteroids and quickly noticed unwanted side effects, including bloating and high blood pressure.

"I was on high doses of steroids, and I felt like I was spiraling," Jake recalls. "My blood pressure shot up, and my weight ballooned. I knew I needed to make a change."

With the guidance of a nutritionist, Jake switched to a plant-based diet that emphasized anti-inflammatory foods. He started incorporating more fruits, vegetables, and whole grains, while cutting back on processed foods and sugar. He also made it a point to add more omega-3-rich foods like flaxseeds, walnuts, and chia seeds to his meals.

"Honestly, the change wasn't easy at first. I loved fast food, and I didn't think I could give it up. But after a few weeks, I began to feel the difference. My blood pressure dropped, and the bloating subsided. My doctor was able to lower my steroid dose, and I had more energy throughout the day."

For Jake, diet has become an essential part of his treatment plan, and he continues to manage his PMR symptoms while balancing the demands of his job. "If you're thinking about trying dietary changes, go for it. It's one of the best decisions I've made."

Sarah's Story: Early Diagnosis and Proactive Changes

Sarah, 55, was diagnosed with PMR early on after experiencing severe pain that made it hard to lift her arms. She was put on steroids but wanted to take a proactive approach to avoid long-term dependency on medication.

"I'm very health-conscious, and I didn't want to rely on

medication if I didn't have to," Sarah says. "So I started looking into how diet could help manage the inflammation."

Sarah chose to follow an anti-inflammatory, whole-foods-based diet with a strong focus on omega-3 fatty acids, lean protein sources like fish and legumes, and lots of vegetables. She also made a conscious effort to include more turmeric and ginger, known for their anti-inflammatory properties.

"It was a learning process, but I stuck with it, and I started to see results. My pain was more manageable, and my doctor gradually lowered my steroid dosage. I don't think I would have been able to wean off them as quickly if I hadn't changed my diet."

Sarah continues to eat a balanced diet that emphasizes anti-inflammatory foods. While she still experiences flare-ups from time to time, she feels empowered to manage her condition. "Diet isn't a magic bullet, but it's a huge part of the equation."

Margaret's Story: A Holistic Approach to Long-Term Management

At 70, Margaret has lived with PMR for nearly 10 years. Her condition initially left her bedridden, struggling to get through the day. Over time, she realized that managing PMR required a holistic approach.

"Steroids helped, but I couldn't shake the side effects. My weight kept creeping up, and I was constantly fatigued. It wasn't just about the pain anymore—it was my overall health."

Margaret began to overhaul her diet, incorporating foods known to fight inflammation. She started making smoothies with greens, berries, and flaxseed for breakfast and chose fish or legumes for dinner. She cut out processed foods and sugary snacks, replacing them with nuts and fresh fruit.

"I still have bad days, but I can tell the difference when I'm eating clean. I feel less bloated, and my joints aren't as stiff. My energy levels are higher, and I'm even able to go for walks again."

Margaret continues to work with a healthcare team to manage her symptoms through a combination of diet, medication, and physical therapy. "PMR is a part of my life, but it doesn't define me anymore. Making changes to my diet has helped me regain control."

David's Story: Finding Balance

David, 60, was diagnosed with PMR after months of chronic pain and sleepless nights. As an active man who enjoyed outdoor activities, he found his world shrinking as the condition took hold.

"I couldn't do the things I loved anymore," David shares. "Every time I moved, it hurt. I was losing my sense of self."

After starting corticosteroids, David knew he had to address the weight gain and bloating. He also wanted to support his body through dietary changes. He adopted a Mediterranean-style diet, focusing on whole grains, lean proteins, and plenty of fruits and vegetables. Olive oil, salmon, and nuts became staples in his meals.

"Over time, I found a balance. The combination of the right foods and medication has given me a better quality of life. I'm not 100%, but I'm better."

David encourages others with PMR to explore dietary interventions. "Every little change helps. It's about finding what works for you."

In Summary

These personal stories highlight the power of dietary changes in managing PMR. While each person's journey is unique, the common thread is that adopting an anti-inflammatory diet can significantly improve quality of life. By incorporating foods that reduce inflammation and avoiding those that exacerbate symptoms, individuals with PMR can take charge of their health and manage their condition more effectively. These stories illustrate that, while the path may be challenging, it is possible to live well with PMR by making conscious dietary and lifestyle choices.

17. Conclusion

As we reach the conclusion of this book, it's crucial to emphasize not only the importance of managing polymyalgia rheumatica (PMR) through diet but also the broader responsibility we bear in making ethical food choices. While the primary focus of this book has been the Modern Polymyalgia Diet, and how dietary choices can play a significant role in managing inflammation and enhancing quality of life for those living with PMR, the wider implications of our food choices cannot be overlooked.

Why are ethical food choices important, particularly for those managing chronic inflammatory diseases such as polymyalgia rheumatica? In addition to supporting personal health, the foods we choose impact the environment, animal welfare, and the global economy. The rise in popularity of health-focused diets, including the Mediterranean diet, has sparked conversations about the ethical considerations surrounding the production and consumption of food.

A Mediterranean-style diet has been shown to reduce inflammation, which is crucial for managing PMR. However, the benefits of these diets go beyond symptom management—they also offer an opportunity to reflect on how we approach eating in an ethical and responsible manner.

The Connection Between Food Choices and Ethical Eating

Ethical eating involves being mindful of how our food choices affect the world around us. It requires considering the environmental, social, and animal welfare impacts of the foods we consume. Ethical food choices reflect a commitment to reducing harm wherever possible, ensuring that our diets contribute positively not only to our health but to the health of the planet and the well-being of others.

Incorporating whole foods, fruits, vegetables, legumes, nuts, and seeds into your diet, as recommended for managing PMR, can support your health. But it is equally important to be mindful of the sustainability of the food production systems behind these foods. Here, we examine the key ethical considerations that should shape how we approach our dietary choices.

Environmental Impact

The environmental footprint of food production is one of the most significant ethical concerns in modern agriculture. Large-scale farming practices can have devastating consequences on ecosystems. The overuse of natural resources like land and water, soil degradation, deforestation, and excessive greenhouse gas emissions are just a few examples of how food production impacts the environment.

For example, the production of certain foods, even those commonly considered healthy, such as lean meats and fish, has ethical implications. While lean meats are often recommended for their low fat content, their mass production contributes to environmental degradation. Overgrazing, pollution from animal waste, and methane emissions from livestock are all factors that strain our planet. Similarly, the growing demand for fish as a source of lean protein has led to overfishing, threatening marine biodiversity and disrupting ocean ecosystems.

Ethical food choices, therefore, require consumers to be mindful of how their food is produced. Supporting sustainable agricultural practices, such as organic farming and buying locally grown produce, can help mitigate some of the negative environmental impacts of food production. In the context of the Modern Polymyalgia Diet, this might mean choosing plant-based proteins over animal-based ones or opting for sustainably sourced fish when including seafood in your meals.

Social Impact

Our food choices also have far-reaching social implications. The way food is produced, processed, and distributed can affect local communities and economies. Labor practices in the food industry often come under scrutiny, particularly in relation to wages and working conditions. The workers involved in harvesting, processing, and transporting food often face poor working conditions, low wages, and exploitation. Additionally, the overconsumption of imported foods can undermine local agricultural industries, particularly in developing countries where small-scale farmers rely on their local markets for sustenance.

To make socially responsible food choices, consumers can prioritize purchasing foods that are produced under fair trade practices and support local economies by buying from nearby farmers' markets or community-supported agriculture programs. This is not only a more ethical approach but also ensures fresher, more nutrient-dense produce—further supporting the goals of managing PMR through nutrition.

Animal Welfare

For those managing PMR, ethical considerations surrounding animal welfare should not be ignored. The Modern Polymyalgia Diet encourages the inclusion of lean meats, but it is important to consider the ethical implications of animal farming. Industrial farming practices often involve the use of hormones and antibiotics to enhance growth and production, contributing to significant ethical concerns regarding the treatment of animals.

Furthermore, confined animal feeding operations (CAFOs) can cause immense suffering, with animals living in overcrowded, unsanitary conditions. The ethical treatment of animals should be a priority when making food choices, and consumers can make a difference by choosing humanely raised, grass-fed, or organic animal products.

Alternatively, as more research supports the health benefits of plant-based diets for inflammatory diseases like PMR, incorporating more plant-based proteins into your diet can be both an ethical and health-conscious choice.

Navigating Ethical Grey Areas in the Mediterranean Diet

While the Mediterranean diet is widely recognized for its health benefits, particularly in reducing inflammation and improving cardiovascular health, it is not without ethical challenges. The overconsumption of certain foods that are staples of this diet—such as olive oil, wine, and certain nuts—can have detrimental effects on the environment.

For example, olive oil production, when intensified to meet global demand, can lead to soil degradation and water scarcity in the regions where olives are grown. Similarly, the cultivation of nuts like almonds requires vast amounts of water, further straining environmental resources. The key to navigating these ethical grey areas is to consume these foods in moderation and to support sustainable farming practices whenever possible.

Practical Steps for Ethical Eating

In light of these ethical considerations, you might wonder what steps you can take to make a positive impact. Here are some practical tips to guide you in making more ethical food choices:

1. **Educate Yourself**: Understanding the environmental, social, and animal welfare implications of your food choices is the first step toward making more ethical decisions. Stay informed about the sources of your food and the practices involved in its production.

2. **Support Sustainable Farming**: Whenever possible, choose organic and sustainably produced foods. Look for certifications such as USDA Organic, Fair Trade, and Marine Stewardship Council (MSC) to ensure your food is sourced ethically.

3. **Buy Local**: Supporting local farmers not only reduces the carbon footprint associated with transporting food over long distances but also helps local economies thrive. Fresh, locally grown produce often contains more nutrients and flavor, further supporting your health.

4. **Reduce Meat Consumption**: Opting for plant-based proteins more often can reduce the environmental and ethical impact of your diet. If you do consume meat, choose grass-fed, organic, or humanely raised options.

5. **Avoid Overconsumption**: Even healthy foods can have negative consequences when consumed in excess. Moderation is key to both personal health and environmental sustainability.

6. **Choose Seasonal Foods**: Eating with the seasons ensures that your food is fresher and more in harmony with local ecosystems, reducing the need for artificial growing practices and long-distance transportation.

7. **Advocate for Change**: As consumers, we have the power to

influence the food industry through our purchasing choices. By choosing ethically produced foods and supporting companies that prioritize sustainability, we send a message that ethical practices are important to us.

Final Thoughts

In conclusion, managing polymyalgia rheumatica through diet is about more than just reducing inflammation and alleviating symptoms. It is an opportunity to rethink how we approach food, ensuring that our choices support not only our own health but the health of the planet and the well-being of others. Ethical food choices are an essential part of the Modern Polymyalgia Diet, and incorporating these considerations into your daily life can lead to both personal and collective benefits.

As we look ahead, it's important to recognize that making ethical choices is a continuous journey. There is no perfect diet or perfect solution, but through conscious effort, we can reduce the negative impacts of our food choices and contribute to a healthier, more sustainable future for all.

Thank you for joining us on this journey toward better health and a better world. I hope that this book has provided you with not only valuable dietary insights for managing PMR but also the tools to make informed, ethical decisions in your everyday life.

Sincerely,

Cheryl White, MAT

Sandra Faix, PhD

Appendix A: Food Substitutes

Making conscious substitutions in your diet is key to reducing inflammation and managing PMR symptoms effectively. Below are suggestions for replacing common inflammatory foods with healthier, anti-inflammatory alternatives.

Carbohydrates

Instead of refined carbohydrates like **white bread** or **white rice**, choose whole grain alternatives:

- **Whole grain bread, quinoa,** or **brown rice** are excellent substitutes, rich in fiber and nutrients that help regulate blood sugar and reduce inflammation.

- For pasta, replace it with **whole grain pasta, quinoa,** or **sweet potatoes,** which offer lower glycemic index options to help stabilize blood sugar levels.

Proteins

Protein plays an essential role in your diet, but certain proteins like **red meat** can increase inflammation. Replace them with healthier options:

- Opt for **wild-caught fatty fish** such as **salmon, mackerel,** or **sardines.** These are rich in omega-3 fatty acids, which are powerful anti-inflammatory agents.

●   If you prefer poultry, choose **free-range turkey** or **chicken**, which are healthier and ethically produced.

●   For a plant-based option, try **lentils, chickpeas,** or **tempeh**. These legumes are protein-packed and help reduce inflammation while supporting overall health.

Fats

Avoid unhealthy fats like trans fats found in **margarine** or fried foods, and choose healthier fats that reduce inflammation:

●   Replace margarine or **vegetable oil** with **extra virgin olive oil** or **avocado oil**. These oils are rich in monounsaturated fats and antioxidants, supporting heart health and reducing inflammation.

●   Include **nuts** such as **walnuts** or **almonds**, and seeds like **flaxseeds** or **chia seeds**, which are high in omega-3s and are anti-inflammatory.

Dairy

Certain dairy products can contribute to inflammation, so it's important to consider alternatives:

●   Instead of full-fat dairy like **whole milk** or **cheese**, choose **unsweetened almond milk, coconut milk,** or **cashew milk**. These options are dairy-free and often fortified with essential nutrients like calcium.

●   For yogurt, opt for **Greek yogurt**, which contains probiotics that help promote gut health and reduce inflammation, while being lactose-friendly for those sensitive to dairy.

Sugary Beverages

High-sugar drinks contribute to inflammation and insulin

spikes. Replace these with hydrating and anti-inflammatory options:

- Swap **soda, fruit juices**, and sugary beverages for **water, herbal teas**, or **water infused with lemon, cucumber**, or **mint**.

- For a refreshing alternative, try **sparkling water** with a splash of 100% fruit juice for flavor without the sugar overload.

Snacks

Processed snacks are loaded with unhealthy fats, sugars, and additives. Here are better options:

- Instead of **chips, crackers**, or **packaged snacks**, try **raw nuts** like **almonds** or **walnuts**, or a mix of **seeds**.

- **Fresh vegetable sticks** (carrots, cucumbers, celery) with a side of **hummus** or **guacamole** make for a nutritious, anti-inflammatory snack.

- Choose **fresh fruits** like berries, which are packed with antioxidants, or **dried fruits** like apricots (in moderation, due to their sugar content).

Cooking Methods

Cooking methods can also influence the inflammatory potential of your meals. Here are healthier alternatives to frying:

- Instead of **fried foods**, bake, grill, or steam your vegetables and proteins. **Roasting** can also bring out natural flavors while maintaining a healthier fat profile.

- **Slow-cooking** or **pressure cooking** can be great ways to maintain the nutrients in vegetables and lean meats without adding inflammatory oils.

By integrating these anti-inflammatory food substitutes into your diet and choosing ethically sourced options like **wild-caught fish** and **free-range poultry**, you can manage PMR symptoms more effectively while also considering the broader environmental and ethical implications of your diet.

Appendix B: Cooking Tips for Beginners

If you're new to cooking or feel overwhelmed by meal prep, these simple tips can help you ease into the Modern PMR Diet while enjoying delicious, nutritious meals. Don't worry—cooking healthy doesn't have to be complicated!

1. Start Simple with One-Pan Meals

One-pan or one-pot meals are beginner-friendly, easy to clean up, and you can add a variety of anti-inflammatory foods. For example, a sheet pan dinner of salmon and roasted vegetables drizzled with olive oil is simple, nutritious, and quick.

Tip: Preheat your oven to 400°F, place your fish and veggies on a baking sheet, drizzle with olive oil, season with herbs, and bake for 20–25 minutes.

2. Use Pre-Cut or Frozen Veggies

There's no need to chop everything from scratch—many grocery stores offer pre-cut fresh vegetables or frozen options that are just as nutritious. This saves time and effort in meal prep.

Tip: Keep bags of frozen vegetables like spinach, broccoli, or mixed vegetables in your freezer for quick additions to stir-fries, soups, or smoothies.

3. Cook in Batches

Batch cooking is a time-saver for those with busy schedules. Prepare larger portions of anti-inflammatory dishes like soups, stews, or grain bowls on the weekend and store them in the fridge or freezer for easy meals during the week.

Tip: Make a large batch of quinoa or brown rice and use it throughout the week in salads, stir-fries, or as a side dish.

4. Invest in Basic Kitchen Tools

You don't need a fancy kitchen setup to cook nutritious meals. A few simple tools will make a big difference:

- A **good knife** for chopping vegetables

- A **sheet pan** for roasting

- A **blender** for smoothies or soups

- **Measuring spoons** and cups for accurate portioning

Tip: If you enjoy smoothies or soups, consider getting an immersion blender for quick blending with minimal cleanup.

5. Learn to Season with Herbs and Spices

Spices like turmeric, ginger, and garlic have natural anti-inflammatory properties, and they're easy to add to any dish. Fresh herbs like parsley, cilantro, or basil also boost flavor without added calories or salt.

Tip: Experiment with seasoning blends, like Italian herbs (basil, oregano) for Mediterranean dishes or curry spices (cumin, coriander, turmeric) for Indian-inspired meals.

6. Don't Be Afraid of Shortcuts

Shortcuts like using rotisserie chicken (free-range and ethically sourced), canned low-sodium beans, or pre-made salad mixes can make meal prep more manageable, especially on busy nights.

Tip: If you're using canned beans, make sure to rinse them under cold water to reduce sodium content before adding them to dishes like salads or stews.

7. Create Easy Salad and Snack Prep

Prepare snacks and salads ahead of time to stay on track. Wash and chop veggies, then store them in containers for easy access. Pair them with hummus, nuts, or a homemade vinaigrette for a quick, anti-inflammatory snack or meal.

Tip: Build a salad in layers for freshness. Start with sturdy greens like kale or spinach at the bottom, then add other ingredients like cucumbers, cherry tomatoes, nuts, and top with your protein just before eating.

8. Grill or Bake Instead of Frying

Grilling or baking foods keeps them healthier by reducing the amount of unhealthy fats. Whether it's fish, vegetables, or poultry, these methods ensure you retain the nutrients without extra calories or inflammation-inducing trans fats.

Tip: When grilling or baking fish, add a squeeze of lemon and a sprinkle of your favorite herbs (like dill or thyme) to enhance the flavor without needing extra sauces.

9. Plan for Leftovers

Whenever you cook, make extra servings and store them in airtight containers. You can use leftovers for a different meal, like adding roasted vegetables to a quinoa salad or turning leftover grilled chicken into a wrap with whole wheat tortillas and veggies.

Tip: Label your containers with dates so you know when to use them, and refrigerate or freeze as needed.

ABOUT THE AUTHORS

Cheryl White has been a dedicated health science writer for more than 30 years. With an undergraduate degree in Health Sciences and two master's degrees, Cheryl has spent her career educating others on health-related topics. Her vast experience spans topics from chronic conditions to the latest advancements in medical science. Cheryl's passion for helping people live healthier lives comes through in her writing, making complex health issues understandable and accessible for all readers.

Sandra Faix, PhD, is a certified nutritionist and lecturer with a decade of experience in the field of human dietetics. After earning her PhD in human dietetics, Sandra has focused her career on teaching and helping individuals make informed, nutritious choices. As a nutrition expert, she understands the intricate role that diet plays in managing chronic conditions like polymyalgia rheumatica (PMR) and works to create practical, accessible nutrition advice. Sandra's research-driven insights guide readers in making sustainable and healthful dietary choices to improve overall well-being.

www.ingramcontent.com/pod-product-compliance
Lightning Source LLC
Chambersburg PA
CBHW061400250726

48657CB00004B/1580